TEXTURED TRESSES

The Ultimate Guide to Maintaining and Styling Natural Hair

DIANE DA COSTA

With Paula T. Renfroe

A Fireside Book
Published by Simon & Schuster
NEW YORK LONDON TORONTO SYDNEY

FIRESIDE
Rockefeller Center
1230 Avenue of the Americas
New York, NY 10020

FIRESIDE and colophon are registered trademarks
of Simon & Schuster, Inc.

For information regarding special discounts for bulk purchases,
please contact Simon & Schuster Special Sales at
1-800-456-6798 or business@simonandschuster.com

Designed by Joy O'Meara Battista and Chris Welch

Manufactured in the United States of America

3   5   7   9   10   8   6   4

Library of Congress Cataloging-in-Publication Data
Da Costa, Diane.
Textured tresses : the ultimate guide to maintaining and styling natural hair /
Diane Da Costa, with Paula T. Renfroe.
p.   cm.
Includes bibliographical references and index.
1. Hairdressing of Blacks.   2. Hair—Care and hygiene.
I. Renfroe, Paula T.   II. Title.

TT972.D33   2004
646.7'24'08996073—dc22   2004045344

ISBN 0-7432-3550-9

311703

Dedicated to Women of Strength
My Adoring Mother, Naomi Da Costa,
and
In Loving Memory of
Sicily Da Costa
and
Cora Francis

Creative Team

Author
Diane Da Costa

Co-Writer
Paula T. Renfroe

Cover
Creative Direction
    Photography—Roberto Ligresti (Diane Da Costa),
       George Larkins (models), Pieter M. van Hattem
       (Roy Hargrove)
    Makeup—Sam Fine
    Hair Styling—Diane Da Costa
    Hair Color—Rudy/Artista Salon, NYC

Production
Creative Direction
Todd Wilson for Chemistry Lab, NYC (photo shoot)
Hollis King, VP, Verve Music Group, Consultant

Production Assistants
Pamela Greenidge, Angela Jones, Ekem Merchant, Tammi Cobbs,
   Victoria Powell

Photography
Kwaku Alston—Blair Underwood (Foreword)
George Larkins—Interior
Niya Bascom—Chapter 16: Improvisation

Contributing Photographers
Marc Baptiste, Matthew Jordan Smith, Matthew Rolston, Peter
   Ogilvie, Jon Peden, Jack Guy, Mark Higashino, Vincent Soyez,
   Jimmy Bruch, Preston Thomas, Gregg Routt, Deborah Lopez,
   Barron Claiborne, Jinsey Dauk, Eric von Lockhart

Illustrators
Renaldo Davidson, Renaldo Studios, NYC (afros, Josephine
   Baker)
Alvin Kofi, Bushmen USA (Tehuti Productions), London
   (Massai Warrior)
James Walker—Part 2: Achieve It! (all illustrations)

Hair Artistry—Creative Direction
Diane Da Costa
Jamillah Ferris (assistant)

Contributing Stylists
Dekar Lawson, Dekar Salon, NYC
Ona the Locksmyth, Locksmyths Loc Groomers, Brooklyn, NY
Nene D'diaye, Khamit Kinks, NYC
Renee Cooper, Turning Heads Salon Spa, NYC
Hadiiya Barbel, Studio One, Brooklyn, NY
Ray Issa, Artista Salon Spa, NYC

Makeup Artistry
Ayinde Castro, Debra Martin Agency
Fatima Thomas (M.A.C.)
Natasha Drarnel, Illusions/Click
Valente Frazier, Nikita Houston, Danni Ley, DL.d Reps, NYC
Eric Spearman, Illusions/Click

Wardrobe Stylists
Carlene Ferguson, Mary Lafayette, Kimberly Wilks, Paul Petzy,
    Roderick Studios & Co., Inc.

Wardrobe
Epperson-NYC, Exodus Industrial Clothing, NYC
The Brownstone, Harlem, NY
Phat Farm and Baby Phat, NYC
Minu Hu Dres, Atlanta, GA
H & M, NYC

Jewelry
Roderick Studios & Co., Inc., NYC

Accessories
denise kerr designs, Brooklyn, NY (leather rollup styling case)

Models
HBM Models—Jessica deSouza, Nanya Akuka Goodrich, Giovanna
    Leonardo, Nicole Fisiella, Linda Nguyen, Tanya Martinez,
    Shannon Quinton, Nikisha Riley, Tamikko Willis Spica, Denise
    Marie, Emie, Lisa Friend, Freedom Bradley, Freedom Bremner
    (recording artist), Tracy Grant, Alicia Hall, Malonda Richard,
    Chrystal Wong

CREATIVE TEAM

Chapter 13: Textured Hair for the Family
Chelsea and Leon Dorsey, Deidre Poe and Evan Poe Sanders,
　Elizabeth L. Martin, Ed and Taylor Gordon, Genieva Kellam and
　Kara Fowler

Prop Stylist
LaRonce Marshall (Ed Gordon's photo shoot at Platinum
　Investment Properties)

Photo-Shoot Locations
Akwaaba Mansion, Akwaaba Café/Moshan Enterprises,
　Brooklyn, NY
Artista Salon Spa, NYC
Locksmyths Loc Groomers, Brooklyn, NY
Platinum Investment Properties Mansion, NJ
Turning Heads Salon Spa, NYC

Location Coordinator
Kym Norsworthy—Worth Inc. Public Relations
　(Ed Gordon's photo shoot)

Catering
Soul Fixins, NYC
Akwaaba Café, Brooklyn, NY

Advisors and Specialists
Dr. Deborah Simmons (dermatology), private practice, NYC
Dr. Fran Cook-Bolden (dermatology), Director of Ethnic Skin, NYC
Dr. Henry McCurtis (stress management), NYC

Contents

Foreword by Blair Underwood   xiii

Introduction   xvii

PART ONE
PREPPING THE CANVAS
Caring for Your Textured Hair

1   Appreciating the Beauty of Naturally Textured Hair   3

THE BEATITUDES OF LOVING AND ACCEPTING NATURALLY TEXTURED HAIR   12

2   Healthy Hair Is Happy Hair   15

3   Life in a Bottle: Products to Maintain Your Tresses   35

4   Diane's Bag: Tools You Need for Proper Hair Care   45

5   In Harmony: Picking the Right Stylist and Salon   55

6   Shear Perfection: The Necessity for Change via Shaping and Cutting   63

7   Chemically Speaking: Changing God-Given Texture for Manageability and Versatility   71

PART TWO
ACHIEVE IT!
Styling Your Textured Hair

8 Natural Sets and Styles   85

9 Twists and Turns   99

10 Coils and Curls   109

11 Locking and Tightening Up   117

12 Braids and Weaves   131

13 Textured Hair for the Family   143

14 The Aura of Color and Illumination   149

15 Cover Shots   159

16 Improvisation: Glamorous Styles for Men and Women   161

Salon Directory   165

Recommended Products   177

References   179

Art Credits   180

Acknowledgments   185

Index   189

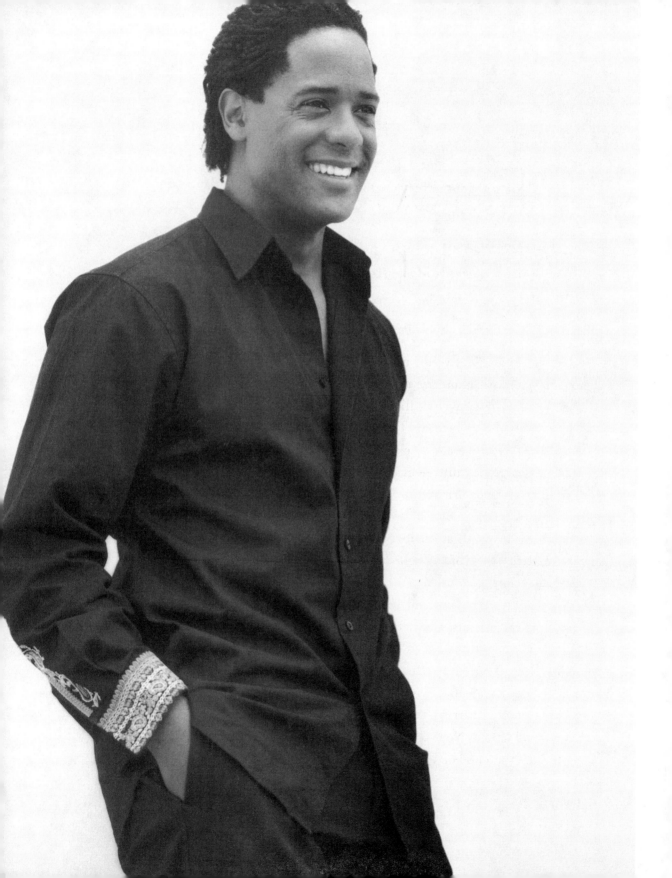

Foreword by Blair Underwood

From a very young age, I knew that I not only possessed a vivid imagination like most children, but also that I never wanted to lose my childlike spirit. A distinct part of me craved make-believe and fantasy. The possibility of opening a book, watching a movie, creating characters in a play, or escaping to magical lands, galaxies, and universes consumed me.

Because I was born into a military family, my siblings and I were raised on a healthy diet of practicality and pragmatism. So, I had a dilemma. How does a child who doesn't want to grow up compromise with other factions of himself that scream, "Be sensible!"? Answer: Become an actor!

Choosing this insane and wonderful business was thankfully sanctioned by my parents, who actually did an outstanding job of balancing our majestic dreams with the mundane realities of the world in which we live. So, off I went in search of as many diverse characters to portray and become as possible. Diversity, versatility, chapter and verse—these were the tools I carried with me when I went off to college to study drama and later to New York in search of a show business career.

As time marched on and more and more jobs came my way, I found myself creating different characters from the inside out (as we were taught in drama school). In other words, finding the inner life first and then building the exterior. I've always enjoyed this layer of the creative process, creating the "look." His wardrobe, walk, speech patterns, etc.—oh yes, and of course, his hair.

Which brings me to Diane Da Costa. I was first introduced to Diane more than a decade ago in Los Angeles. We worked in different areas of the entertainment industry—Diane as a natural hair care specialist and me as an actor. Over the years, I've consulted with Diane numerous times regarding different hairstyles. Whether I was manufacturing locs for the short film *The Second Coming* or sporting twists and cornrows, Diane has been a reliable and dependable source of knowledge and insight. In May 2001 while I was shooting the film *G,* Diane established the "twisted" look for my character. While she had me on "lockdown" in her chair, she launched into a barrage of questions about how men (collectively) and I (individually) felt about hair and women.

In my opinion, a woman's hair is inextricably linked to either her sexuality or, at the very least, a man's perception of her sexuality. Sexual preferences notwithstanding, it is more a question of how she embraces her sexuality and femininity. Does she embrace them? Does she even love herself?

After a long, in-depth interview with my dear friend Diane, I was honored when she asked me to write the Foreword to *Textured Tresses.*

The Follic Symbol

Follicle (fol-i-cle) n. 1. A tiny anatomical cavity or sac <a hair follicle>.

Phallic (fa-lik) adj. derived from the word "phallus." An aspect of the male anatomy commonly used for procreation.

FOREWORD BY BLAIR UNDERWOOD

The Follic Symbol is deliberately sexual in its inference. Hair atop the statuesque creation we call woman speaks to our innermost senses and fundamental nature. It matters not the shape, color, length, or texture. The outgrowth that emerges from the hair follicle is ofttimes strong and durable. In other cases the actual hair may be fine and threadlike. Whatever the case, the hair will eventually take shape and form a life of its own.

As "man cannot live by bread alone," the true essence and beauty of a woman cannot be attained by great hair alone. Therefore, man cannot fall in love or make love to a great hairdo alone. The search for inner beauty and substance must always take precedence, and then the physical and/or outward attributes will always resonate at a higher frequency.

Whether the hair subtly frames the face to which our eyes are drawn or mischievously taunts us as it dangles and caresses her cheeks while she peeks from behind it, it makes no difference. Whether the coarse, sensual coils we've named afro boldly adorn her regal visage or braids in the ancient styles of Africa cascade down her back as she sashays through her day, it makes no difference. Her strands may be bone-straight, unable to hold the coveted "curl of the day," hanging low and mesmerizing as they waft in the wind. Maybe hers are locs that are anything but *dreadful.* Akin to the mighty lion's mane, her locs conjure images of strength, confidence, endurance, dominance, vitality, and fertility.

The look, feel, and length are irrelevant. As men, it makes us no never mind. We thank our Creator for not only creating you (our better half), but for equipping you with the gift of The Follic Symbol—that strand of hair that, collectively with like strands, hypnotizes, fascinates, soothes, teases, taunts, enthralls, and captivates. Thank God for the Follic Symbol!

—*Blair Underwood*

Introduction

t's an era of rebirth and what do you see? Take a close look. Textured hairstyles are everywhere. Sexy cornrows and bushy afros work the runways of Paris and Milan, the sidewalks of both Tokyo and Philadelphia, as well as the sweaty courts of the NBA and WNBA. Locs and twists adorn the heads of your favorite celebrities. It's no wonder. Textured Hair is Beautiful Hair!

Most women desire something other than what they already have, especially when it comes to our own hair. We want longer, fuller, thicker hair with more manageability, control, flexibility, and options. Well, I have one word for you—texture. Texture will give you everything you're seeking and then some. Textured hair allows you to have it all.

Sometimes reinvention is the mother of invention. With that said, I'd like to offer a new spin on something we've known all along. Texture is what you can see with your eyes and feel to the touch. Texture, as it relates to hair, refers to the straightness or curliness of the hair's surface, yet it is also the softness, roughness, or coarseness, if you will. Texture is straight, wavy, curly, very curly, and tightly coiled hair, too. Cornrows, afros, locs, twists, braids, and knots are styles with texture. Texture is what we all desire and want.

No longer must we apologize for our textured hair. Instead we should celebrate, love, and appreciate our God-given texture. This begins with

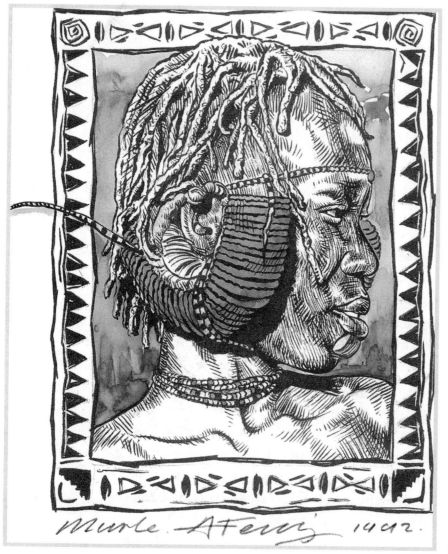

MASSAI WARRIOR

taking pride in acknowledging that certain styles originated from specific regions in Africa. The Samburu people of the Massai Tribe in Kenya and Tanzania wore locs first.

The Samburus were herders who lived above the equator. Before becoming warriors, the young boys prepared their hair with ochre, a red clay mask. The boys would fling their ochre-colored hair in the face of girls they wanted to meet and the girls would flirt back with the young warriors.

The soft, wavy, textured hair like that of the cover model Waris Dirie is common in her homeland of Ethiopia. West Africa is the birthplace of Senegalese twists and many braided styles.

Our flair with textured hair in America is nothing new. It's merely a rediscovery. In the roaring 20s, the Marcel curls and waves were worn by practically every woman, both black and white. In fact, when Cicely Tyson needed to portray a character who wore Marcel waves during that era for the movie *Hoodlum*, she turned to Helen Graine Faulk, the oldest living cosmetologist at the time in Ohio. Apparently no one on the set knew how to create the waves without relaxing Ms. Tyson's natural hair (which was completely unacceptable to her). Ms. Faulk consulted with Cicely Tyson and created the beautiful waves by pressing her hair and using Marcel irons.

Think back to the shiny, slicked-back ponytail of the lovely Billie Holiday in the 40s, the luscious waves of Dorothy Dandridge in the 40s and 50s, and the fierce yet sexy afro of Pam Grier in the 70s.

Michaela Angela Davis, former editor-in-chief of *Honey* magazine, remembers getting her hair cornrowed and rocking afros in the 70s. "When the other kids in high school wore relaxers, I wore braids," says Michaela. "In D.C., there were braiders at the museum on Saturdays and Sundays braiding hair."

Remember the long loc extensions of Lisa Bonet in the 80s? Let's not forget Janet Jackson's Casamas braids in *Poetic Justice*. Many braiders can attest to clients, both regular and new, requesting the "Janet Jackson braids." And no one can deny the impact of Brandy's individual braids worn in various lengths, widths, and styles during the 90s.

Today we see the vibrant wavy hair of Tracee Ellis Ross on UPN's *Girlfriends*, the exotic cornrow extensions of Alicia Keys and Christina

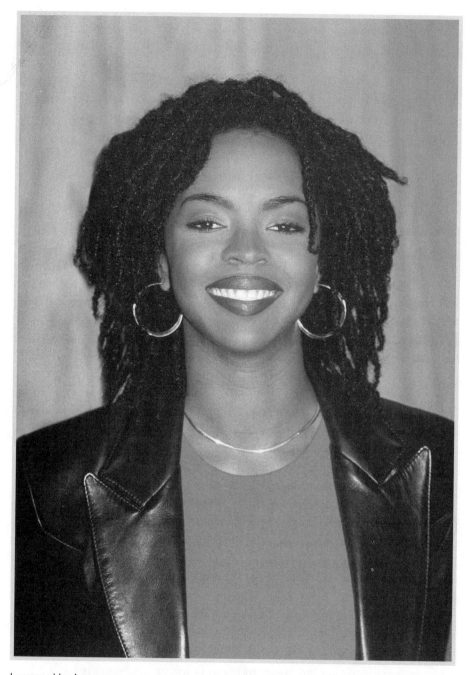

LAURYN HILL'S TRESSES EPITOMIZE THE ENTIRE HAIR MOVEMENT. SHE HAS WORN EVERY
STYLE IMAGINABLE—FROM COILS, BRAIDS, TWISTS, DESIGNER-STYLED LOCS, AND FREE
NATURAL LOCS TO, MOST RECENTLY, A SHORT AND NOW LARGE AFRO.

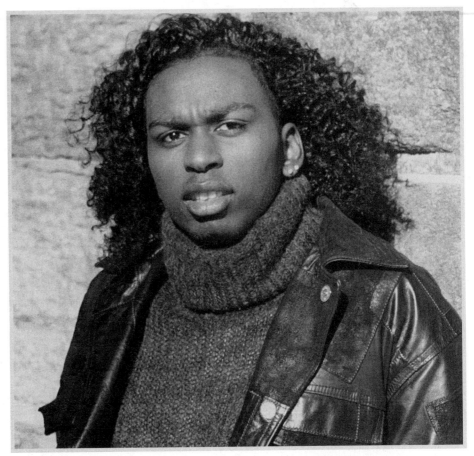

MODEL WITH
TEXTURED HAIR

Aguilera, the sensuous, full, naturally coily 'fros of Lenny Kravitz and Maxwell, and the texturized Caesar worn by Blair Underwood in *Sex and the City*. The possibilities are infinite with Textured Hair.

As a natural hair care specialist, colorist, and precision cutter over the past 15 years, I've seen many of my own textured creations become hair trends, including the Cosmicloc (a loc extension) that appeared in *Moods* magazine in 1990. In the early 90s, while working with model/owner Peggy Dillard of Turning Heads, one of the top-rated natural hair salons in New York City, I got my first big break. *Essence* magazine called the salon to request a style that I called the "Twist Out." Since then my work has appeared on their covers and in their fashion and beauty pages. I've also had the privilege of being the Hair and Beauty Advisor of *Heart & Soul* magazine as well as the first Hair Editor for *Honey* magazine. However, one of my greatest accomplishments was creating and owning Dyaspora Salon and Spa in New York City. This inspiring, trend-setting salon was created to bring artists together in different forums, such as book signings by authors and original artwork showings by painters, where clients would be pampered in a relaxed, cozy environment. It had been my dream since the day I first entered Robert Fiance Hair Design Institute in New York City, just two years after graduating from Pace University with a bachelor's degree in Business Administration and Marketing. I birthed many young, talented stylists, many of whom went on to open their very own salons.

I firmly believe that it is my calling to educate both consumers and professionals with this informative and inspirational natural/textured hairstyling guide that you hold in your very hands. I am an artist at heart and hair is my first canvas. My color tint brush, my shears, and my hands are my tools. I prep the canvas (your hair) before I lay the foundation for every style, then sketch the style that I create for all textures. The goal is to achieve the look. The maintenance serves as the sketch, the plan.

Many of my clients say that I'm a hairstylist to the stars. They say I have magic hands. But if I could perform any trick, it would be to help you rediscover and fall in love with your textured hair, be it straight, wavy, curly, or tightly coiled. Learning to love your textured hair and truly loving yourself go hand in hand. Trust me, I know from personal experience.

As a child I didn't fully appreciate what beautiful textured hair I had. My hair was thick, curly, and naturally long, but I wanted more manageability. I wanted it straighter, so I tried to roller-set my natural hair. That didn't work. It left my hair puffy and out of control.

Like many of you, I still vividly remember my grandmother pressing

INTRODUCTION

my hair. My cousins and I would line up one by one in her kitchen and wait for our turn to get our hair straightened by my grandmother. She pressed each and every one of our heads. My hair was bone straight with tons of oil, and it took quite a few hours to accomplish this task.

As I grew older I learned to care for my own hair. To the surprise of no one, at 15, I became the hairstylist for the entire family—cutting, styling, braiding, plaiting, and creating coils with a wide-tooth comb.

Like many of you, I've sported every relaxed hairstyle imaginable—short and long bobs, straight, and asymmetrical, and in practically every color, too! You name it, I wore it and loved it. Yet it was always in the back of my mind to lock my hair.

In 1986, after one full year of contemplation, I decided to shed my relaxed hair and go natural. I wanted to explore and experiment with the God-given texture of my hair. Instead of locking right away, I went to Kinapps, a renowned hair salon I'd read about in *Essence,* to cut off eight inches of my relaxed hair. As I looked in the mirror and watched Dexter, the barber, gather his shears, I reassured him continuously that this was indeed what I wanted. Dexter was still reluctant. He didn't want me to cut off my thick head of hair, but I insisted. I finally won, though he actually ended up leaving some relaxed hair in the front. Later I would cut it all off.

As I watched him cut my straight hair off inch by inch, it was simultaneously jarring and liberating. Waves of relaxed hair fell past my shoulder and onto the floor, while curly new growth peeked out at my roots.

My boyfriend at the time was shocked and hated it. Quite honestly, it took me a couple of weeks to adjust. But I had made up my mind that I wanted my hair natural and I wanted to lock it. I didn't simply adjust. I made the shift and fell in love with my texture. I began a wonderful, brand-new relationship with my textured hair and we've been in love ever since.

"Textured Hair allows you flexibility and versatility whether worn natural or relaxed," says celebrity stylist Oscar James. Accepting and loving your hair texture will enable you to try all textured hairstyles, providing you with versatility and options. Believe me, I've tried practically every textured hairstyle too, including Caesars; short, medium, and long cuts; braids (micros, cornrows, Cherokee, individuals); coils; twists; Senegalese twists; the Twist Out; flat twists; locs (crimped, rolled, rodded, and colored from black to blonde); and Genilocs. Not only have I had my hair done by African hair braiders, but I've also experimented with fusion and interlocking weaves. Now I don't care whether my hair is long or short. My only concern is that my hair is healthy, shiny, and manageable. If I want longer hair I just add braid extensions. I no longer have to overprocess or over–blow-dry and neither do you. Options, options, we all have options.

We are living in a hair movement. So many of us are wearing our hair natural and free. We should really understand what a privilege it is to be able to wear natural styles in all walks of life. Not long ago, textured styles were viewed as political or unprofessional. Our natural hair pioneers like Sonia Sanchez, Angela Davis, and Nikki Giovanni wore textured styles and were often prejudged and sometimes shunned. However, today we see our people in any profession sporting locs, braids, and twists with much more assuredness and much less retribution.

In *Sisters of the Yam*, the renowned author bell hooks emphasizes the importance of artists like Lauryn Hill, who is often compared to Tracy Chapman, "not only because her music is deep and compelling, but because she has broken new ground in representing a black beauty aesthetic that is rarely depicted positively in this society." Continues hooks: "To see her pictures on album covers, billboards, posters, and in magazines affirms that one does not have to be light-skinned with straight hair and thin nose to be regarded as beautiful."

Textured hair has become more acceptable across the board with grooming, styling, and fashion. Your natural hair is a reflection of who you are. Wear your textured tresses proudly as you walk down the street, as you interview for that position, as you graduate magna cum laude. If you accept yourself, exude confidence, dress well, and are well spoken, there's nothing that can stop you from achieving what is rightfully yours. Your hair will not limit you. Believe in yourself—in all that you are and what you stand for—and you will surely prevail. The road isn't always smooth, but our sisters have paved the way so that we may wear our tresses with dignity and style no matter our path.

"Today it's style," says Bethann Hardison, a former model and one of the initiators of the natural hair movement on the runways of Paris and New York. "You don't have to think twice about it," the owner of Bethann Management continues. "You can have a plus-size woman selling house products on a television commercial and she can wear dreadlocks, or a handsome man on a soap opera and he's wearing dreads. You can see someone with pointy, spiky hair selling teenage products. They're all just reflecting the market. . . . It's giving the market what it's reflecting."

Locs, braids, twists, and fades have exploded onto the mainstream pop culture scene. These and other textured styles like cornrows and knots adorn the heads not only of African Americans, but other ethnic groups as well. These stylish 'dos are wowing the readers of the hippest magazines and viewers of the hottest music videos and movies.

I remember walking out of my salon one day and spotting a young Japanese man with the most beautifully groomed locs I had ever seen on an Asian guy. They were small, even, and tightly groomed. His hair was very straight, so at least two inches of new growth weren't locked yet. This is quite common with straight hair. Sister or Brother locs can be achieved on this hair texture by using a tool to interweave hair directly to the scalp for tighter results and completely locking to the scalp. Or the hair can be braided every time the locs are groomed to get a consistent and tight look at the roots. Still, it was such a fabulous job even with the looseness at the scalp. When I inquired about his locs, he said that his Japanese hair stylist and friend, who now resides in New York, did his hair. I wasn't surprised that the influence of African people had reached the far corners of the earth. Wearing textured styles, as well as performing the techniques to achieve them, is really nothing new. This is why I say it is an era of rebirth, of rediscovery.

Selwyn Seyfu Hinds, author of *Gunshots in My Cook-Up,* is not surprised by the allure of textured hair to other groups "for the same reason that folk have always been drawn to the cultural product of black people," he offers. "Our walk, talk, music, fashion sense, hair . . . black cool, black style, is a food devoured by a mainstream looking to escape its own shackles of tradition and sameness."

Hinds, the former editor-in-chief of *The Source* magazine, also points out that part of it has to do with the way celebrity culture pushes trends.

"Today you have many leading figures in sports and entertainment—Allen Iverson, Lauryn Hill, Jill Scott, etc.—who wear natural hairstyles," says Hinds. "So the things that they represent for many people in terms of beauty, talent, and success, these are also the things that become associated with natural hair. At the same time, you've long had a grassroots movement, outside of celebrity adaptation, toward natural hair, which I think began as an outgrowth of the particular black aesthetic consciousness that flowered in urban centers during the late eighties and early nineties. And when celebrity trend meets grassroots movement, then you have a lasting cultural shift."

It's the perfect time for a book like this. Now, more than ever we are celebrating the beauty of our natural hair. But while many more of us are embracing our natural hair texture, we are not well informed on the proper care, maintenance, and styling of our hair in its natural state. Whether your hair texture is straight, wavy, curly, or tightly coiled you can achieve any hair texture and any textured style. Coloring, shaping, and styling your natural hair will create dimension and depth. You can even enhance texture with multidimensional coloring or texturizing techniques via shaping and cutting. To create dimensional texture on natural hair, consider locs, braids, twists, and free natural sets. Women of color should certainly take advantage of the products, tools, and techniques that assist us in experiencing the virtually endless realm of possibilities our hair texture can create. Ultimately, it's all about texture, and about loving it, living it, appreciating it, and celebrating it with all the glorious options you have with textured hair.

In *Textured Tresses*, I offer you my expertise in using various hair products, tools, and techniques that work specifically well with textured hair, as well as definitive steps to caring, maintaining, and creating the ultimate hairstyles for textured hair.

You'll discover that your textured hair flows with movement and motion whether it is natural or relaxed. You will learn to explore change with a professional stylist through color options, softeners, relaxers, and shaping. And I can't forget about the importance of choosing the best partner as your hairstylist. Just think, this could be a lifetime adventure and a lifelong relationship. Learn to love and appreciate yourself and your own natural texture. I hope that you will obtain a working knowledge of all textures, whether you want to maintain your natural tresses, lock, or just achieve long-lasting, wavy curls. More important, I pray that you'll come to appreciate the beauty of texture, learn to take care of texture, and enjoy experimenting with texture. I've been working with textured hair for most of my life in every curl pattern that you can imagine. I especially enjoy cutting, coloring, and styling. All three allow me to create and have fun. It's like playtime for me. To make a living doing what you love to do is truly a blessing. By the time you finish reading this book, hopefully you will come to see your hair as your true crown and glory.

PART ONE
PREPPING THE CANVAS

Caring for Your Textured Hair

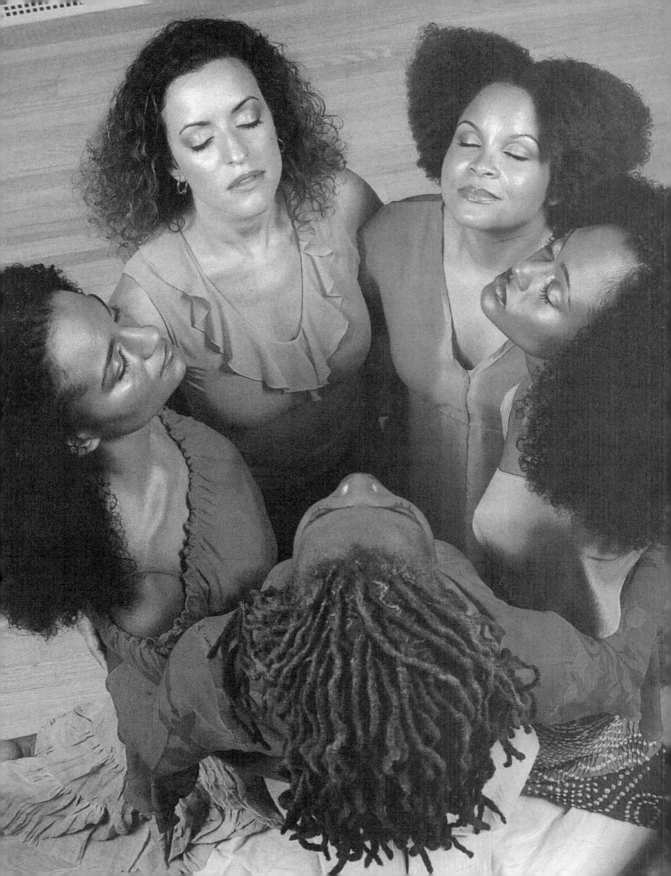

Appreciating the Beauty of Naturally Textured Hair

The universal truth is no matter what nationality we are—African, Asian, or European; Buddhist, Muslim, Christian, or Hebrew; East Indian, Middle Eastern, or descendants or influences of these nations—we all have textured hair. Texture, that's the beauty!

—Diane Da Costa

Let's begin by understanding exactly what texture is. Then you will be better able to identify your own hair's texture. Webster's Dictionary offers three definitions of texture. *1. The surface look or feel of something. 2. The basic makeup of a surface. 3. Distinctive or identifying characteristics.*

Many cosmetology books still refer to texture as only fine or thin, medium, or coarse hair. However, I am proposing that texture is quite simply what you can see and feel. It is the actual straightness or curliness of the hair's surface. Yet, it is also the softness or roughness, the coarseness if you will, of the hair as well.

Textured hair is widely associated with people of color. By "people of color" I mean Africans, African Americans, Caribbeans, Native Americans, Asians, Latinos, East Indians, and every other nonwhite cultural group. Textured hair can achieve any style possible. People of color range in all shades from creamy milk with tightly coiled hair to deep chocolate with straight hair to brown-skinned women with wavy hair to light-skinned women with curly hair.

Dekar Lawson of Dekar Salon in New York City once told me that hair was like either silk or cotton. Well, let's compare hair texture to some inanimate objects for a minute. Hair is like a thin fiber. So straight hair is like silk, which is smooth and sleek. Wavy and loose curly hair is like Persian lambswool, which is springy and moldable. Very curly (spirally) hair is like cotton, which is soft and fluffy. Tightly coiled hair, sometimes called kinky hair, is like wool, which is coarse and lumpy. Remember when the Bible described Jesus' hair as being like wool? The

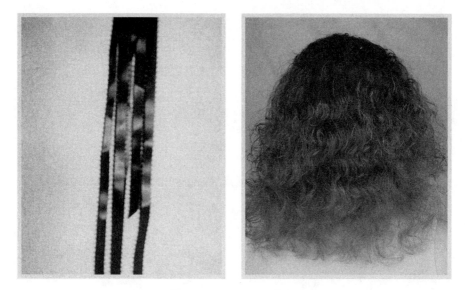

STRAIGHT-WAVE LIKE SILK

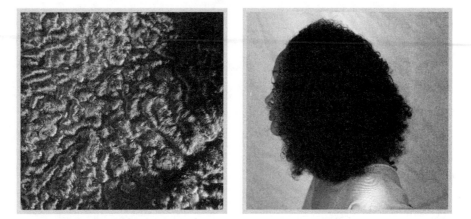

Wavy/loose curly like Persian wool

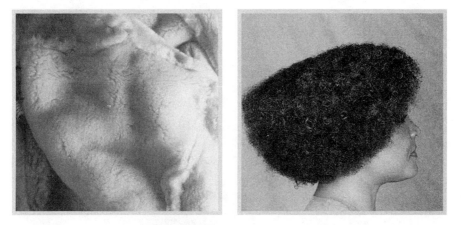

Very curly/spirally like cotton

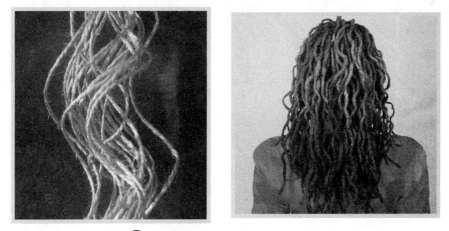

Tightly coiled like coarse wool

Holy Book was talking about the Texture! It is documented in the Bible that both Jesus and Moses had hair of wool.

Samson's hair was said to be the source of his strength, or so everyone believed. However, what really counted was his faith in God and belief that strength really comes from within, the God within you. Loving yourself first will always help you to nurture any style that you or your stylist creates.

There are five basic hair textures that we're dealing with here—straight, wavy, loose curly, very curly, and tightly coiled.

Straight hair, that is, naturally straight hair, is pretty self-explanatory. While Asian and Native-American women tend to have

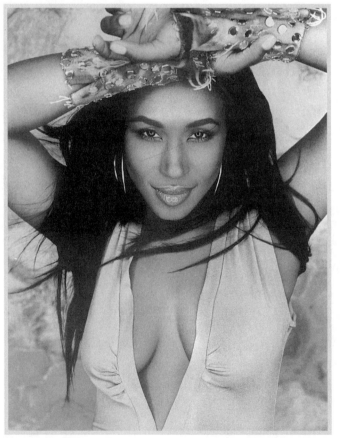

Recording artist Tweet

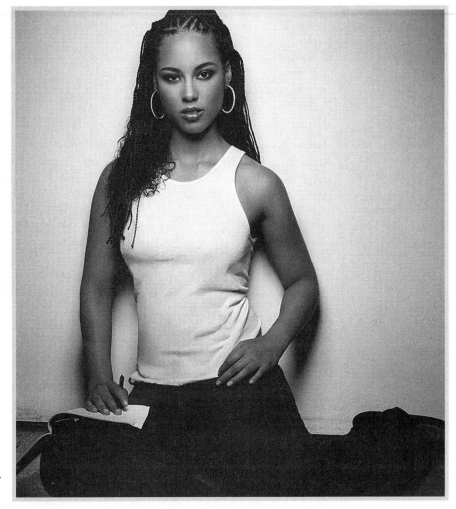

RECORDING ARTIST
ALICIA KEYS

thick, bone-straight hair, most women of color who have "straight" hair have a slight wave pattern. Kimora Lee Simmons, Electra recording artist Tweet, and Alicia Keys are examples of women of color with straight hair. Straight hair is more of a challenge to lock, twist, and braid because of the lack of curl; however, these styles are still very attainable. Though texture is not easily achieved on straight hair, with patience and the right products, tools, and techniques, it most certainly can be accomplished.

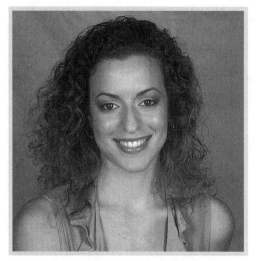

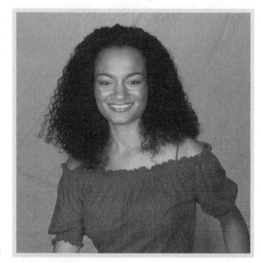

WAVY

Wavy hair, unlike straight hair, has a definite "S" curl pattern, that is, the strands of hair naturally curl into the shape of an "S." Wavy hair tends to be soft, silky, and easy to handle and blow-dry if it is not too thick. Though wavy hair is less challenging to lock, twist, and braid than straight hair, because the wave pattern is so loose the ends must be secured with rods, rubber bands, or molding products. Television host Ananda Lewis has thick, wavy hair as do Latin actress Rosario Dawson and R&B singer Mya.

Loose curly hair is curlier than wavy hair and shapes in the form of a spiral. Loose curly is also easier to add texture to than straight hair. Because loose curly hair has more of a curl pattern than wavy hair, the ends may not need to be secured when twisting, braiding, and locking. The texture of loose curly hair can be changed to a wavy texture with a texturizer (more on texturizing hair in Chapter 7, Chemically Speaking: Changing God-Given Texture for Manageability and Versatility). When brushed and pulled back over a period of time, both wavy and

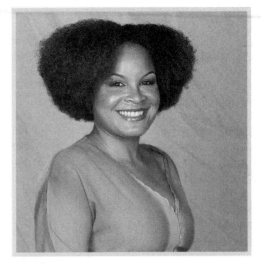

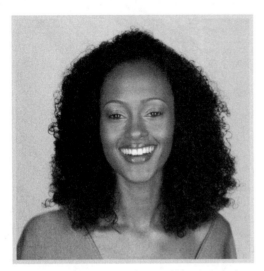

LOOSE CURLY

loose curly hair will become straight. Singers Chilli of the R&B group TLC and Amel Larrieux, formerly of the R&B duo Groove Theory, have loose curly hair.

Very curly hair is very spirally and in humid conditions gets very frizzy. It is ideal for twisting and braiding and very good for locking because of its strong elasticity. Actresses Cree Summer and Tracee Ellis Ross have very curly hair.

Tightly coiled hair has the tightest curl pattern of them all. Tightly coiled hair curls tight to the scalp. Though this type of hair tends to be dry and to snap and break off, with proper care and regular conditioning tightly coiled hair works very well for braiding, cornrowing, twisting, and is the most ideal for locking. The hair texture itself aids in the holding of these styles. Tennis greats Venus and Serena Williams both have tightly coiled hair, as do Vanessa Williams of the television series *Soul Food*, supermodel Alek Wek, and Heather Headley, the singer and Tony Award–winning star of the Broadway musical *Aida*.

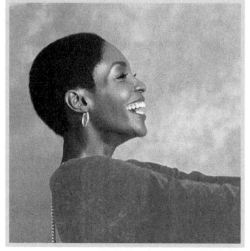

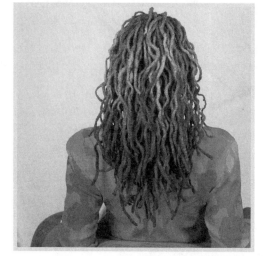

TIGHTLY COILED LOCS

Let's be clear, there is no such thing as good or bad hair, Asian hair, black hair, or white hair. Whatever God has blessed you with is wonderful. You can create wonderful styles with your hair. For the most part, I will concentrate mainly on hair that is naturally free and loose, locs (a permanent, knotted or weaved cylinder form), twists (a two-strand pattern), and braids (a three-strand pattern), all of which are multidimensional and textured. When you touch each of these textured hairstyles you can feel the smoothness or roughness of the surface. Keep in mind that you can achieve a textured hairstyle on hair that is naturally straight or chemically processed. So we can say that waves and curls are textured hair, while coils, braids, and twists are all considered multidimensional textured hairstyles. Versatility, volume, freedom, creativity, and playfulness are just some of the wonderful attributes of texture.

"Texture is versatility," says renowned stylist George Buckner. "I've found that women are freer because they know they can go to the gym. They can go the pool. They can work out. They can walk in the rain and they are not afraid. Before, you were ducking the rain, ducking the water, ducking the pool. You weren't as healthy because you were concerned about your hair. Now with textured hair, you don't have to be concerned with it. Live, love, and be happy!"

Now that you have a better understanding of what texture actually is, we can move on to the most important step—determining your own hair texture.

Let's try this simple exercise. Cut a few strands of hair from different sections of your head: the side, middle, and back. Texture and curl patterns vary throughout the head. People of mixed heritage especially tend to have more than one curl pattern. Next, place the strands on a white piece of paper or napkin. Now compare your hair strands with the individual photos below and find your matching curl pattern.

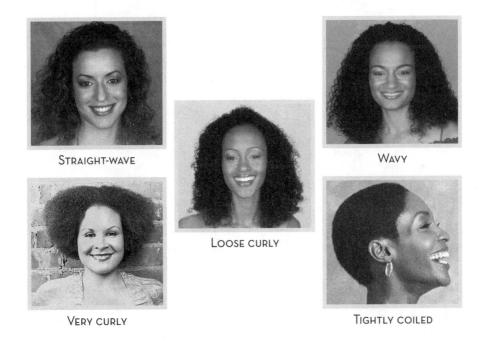

STRAIGHT-WAVE

LOOSE CURLY

WAVY

VERY CURLY

TIGHTLY COILED

Once you make your hair texture determination, we can proceed with creating healthy, happy hair via proper nutrition, exercise, vitamins, products, maintenance, and care of your textured hair.

THE BEATITUDES OF LOVING AND ACCEPTING NATURALLY TEXTURED HAIR

Black women view their hair as a problem. To enjoy black hair, such negative thinking has to be unlearned. And in part we begin to unlearn it by talking to ourselves differently about our hair.

—bell hooks, *Sisters of the Yam*

The beatitudes of loving and accepting your naturally textured hair encompass acceptance, forgiveness, and knowing. Create a meditation area in your home. Find a clean and quiet area with a mirror. Then light incense or scented candles, clear your mind, and recite the Beatitudes below.

Acceptance

- I give thanks and praise to my Father/Mother (Universe) from whom all blessings flow for my (fill in your hair texture: straight, wavy, loose curly, very curly, or tightly coiled) hair.

- I accept the God-given texture I was born with and I promise myself that I will do all that I can to maintain and keep my hair healthy and strong.
- Accept the joy of your natural hair. Bask in the light. Share and don't steal the beauty.
- The beauty of my texture allows me to create any and all styles. I have infinite possibilities and options.
- I love all that I am and all that my hair is, be it short or long.
- I will feed my hair from the inside out through proper nutrition, exercise, and daily maintenance.

Forgiveness

- I forgive myself for abusing my hair and I will do all that I can to nourish it back to a healthy state.
- I will massage my scalp every night to provide blood circulation and promote growth.
- I am giving loving, tender care to my special areas and I see progress each and every day.

Knowing

Give yourself a kiss in the mirror. Style your newfound textured look. Paint your face with as much or as little mascara, oil-free foundation, and lip gloss as you like. Then tell yourself the following:

- Yes, I am beautiful. I am made in the likeness of a perfect, divine me.
- God's got me in the palm of His hand and I walk in the light, shining radiantly with my textured tresses moving fluently and freely.
- Now that I know and understand all about my natural texture, I am among the cognoscenti, those who know. (See References.)

CASSANDRA WILSON, VOCALIST

Healthy Hair
Is Happy Hair

*It is necessary to cultivate the scalp to grow hair as it is to
cultivate the soil to grow a garden.*

—Madam C. J. Walker

Healthy hair is happy hair and everybody wants a head full
of healthy hair, regardless of length or texture. The challenge is knowing how to grow and maintain healthy hair.
The solution is understanding that it starts with nurturing the hair from the inside out. Listen up, ladies: You could buy every
hair product that I personally recommend in this book and it would all
be fruitless if you're not taking care of yourself mentally, physically,
and spiritually. All those old adages hold true—pretty is as pretty does,
beauty is only skin deep, beauty is in the eye of the beholder, and true
beauty comes from within. It's quite simple: If you do not make your
personal health top priority, your hair will show it.

Your hair is a direct reflection of how you feel about yourself and
how well you're nurturing yourself. Our diet and how we care for and

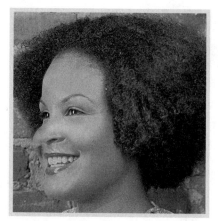

maintain our hair, and what products and/or chemicals we put in our hair will affect the condition of our hair. After our early formative years, it is up to us to maintain the condition of our hair, which is greatly influenced by our diet and lifestyle choices.

"As grownups, many of us look back at childhood years of having our hair combed and braided by other black women as a moment of tenderness and care that was peace-giving and relaxing," says writer bell hooks in *Sisters of the Yam*. "This dimension of sharing in the care of the black female self is necessary in our life and we should seize all opportunity to feel caring hands tending to our hair."

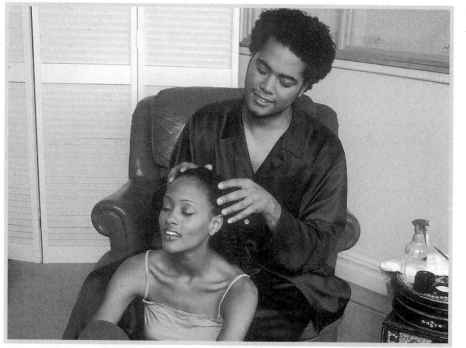

MASSAGING THE
SCALP

Hair Goals for Choosing Healthy Hair

What are your personal hair goals? Taking into consideration your texture, lifestyle, and the present condition of your hair, you could have any style you desire. However, any and every style may not always be what's best for your hair. Knowing which styles are best for your hair is the key to options and versatility. Now, I ask you which comes first, healthy hair or desired style? You make the choice. Here are a few hair goals you should keep in mind for yourself.

- Choose the proper path for your hair texture, whether it is natural or chemically processed.
- Talk to a professional stylist who will guide you through your journey using salon and at-home hair care.
- Although this book will teach you to maintain and style your hair at home, follow a prescribed maintenance program for your tresses that includes:
  - daily maintenance, massaging, and moisturizing.
  - shampoo and conditioning treatments.
  - shaping and trimming on a regular basis.
  - follow-up visits to your stylist.

How Hair Grows

Hair is a thin fiber that consists of protein and minerals. Our hair benefits when we include the proper nutrients in our diet, including protein, fats, minerals, and carbohydrates, according to nutritionist Christina Pirello. Hair relies on the bloodstream for its life and health;

similar to plants, which depend on the nutrients absorbed by the soil. A balanced diet should include protein being seven times that of minerals, and carbohydrates being seven times more than protein. Women who eat a plant-based diet balanced with the above-stated ratios have hair that grows abundantly, according to Pirello. Eating foods of an extremely expansive nature, such as refined sugar, chemicals, strong spices, alcohol, caffeine, nicotine, and tropical fruit can cause the hair to become brittle and delicate, easily damaged and broken. The primary cause of dry hair is the buildup of saturated fat in our bodies, which effectively blocks nutrients and moisture from reaching the hair shaft. Oily hair can be caused by the excessive consumption of saturated fats, and is the precursor to dry hair. Saturated fats are dislodged through the hair shaft, leaving the ends dry and brittle and roots oily.

Hair growth alternates between active and rest periods, with about 85 percent of the hair actively growing and about 15 percent at rest. Hair grows seven times longer than it rests. Autumn and winter are times of the year when the body rests and retains internal warmth. Hair growth slows as the body contracts to conserve energy.

There are three distinct stages of hair growth: the anagen stage, the catagen stage, and the telogen stage. In the anagen stage, hair is growing 85 to 90 percent of the time and the growth period lasts from two to six or seven years. The hair follicle then goes through a slowing-down stage, which is called the catagen stage. Your hair is only growing one percent of the time at this stage. The follicles are getting smaller and smaller and the cells are beginning to die. The telogen stage is the resting stage, and the hair is in this stage 12 to 13 percent of the time. The hair shaft sheds and the follicle may go into a dormant stage. Then it starts all over again. The follicle goes through 15 cycles in a lifetime and then it dies.

"There are certain factors that may contribute to hair growth and loss; however, medically we can't really say why this is the case," says dermatologist Dr. Deborah A. Simmons. "Hormonal factors, growth factors, and chemicals may influence the lack of growth of the follicle or its hair shaft. Genetic factors sometimes play a role and are much more complicated than people can imagine. At any given time all hair on the head grows at different times and at different rates. That's why the hair length on one side of the head may be longer than the other side," explains Dr. Simmons.

What outside factors can have a major effect on the growth cycle? According to Dr. Simmons they include the environment, pollutants, and nutritional influences such as crash diets. Severe anemia caused by iron deficiency can lead to hair loss.

Some vitamins and minerals that have been known to support hair growth or protect the hair follicle from shedding are zinc, vitamin B6, zinc picolinate, and antioxidants, as well as green tea, emu oil from the Australian bird, sesame, and ginger. Though ginger is not recommended for sensitive scalps, odorless garlic is used as an Asian treatment for hair loss.

Essential oils hold the power of ancient medicines from the earth. Their medicinal cleansing properties leave no toxins behind. They cleanse instead of masking odors, according to Valerie Ann Wood's *Complete Book of Essential Oils and Aromatherapy*. Essential oils recommended for hair growth include rosemary, neroli, lavender, geranium, basil, ginger, cedarwood, sage, hyssop, thyme, lemon, grapefruit, cypress, nettles, and goldenseal.

Ancient African, Asian, and Native American Recipes for Hair Growth and Scalp Conditioning

Asian

- Massage equal parts of sesame oil and ginger oil into the scalp for 20 minutes.
- Wrap head with warm towel.
- Shampoo twice.
- Apply leave-in conditioner, then rinse.

Another method:
- Shampoo twice. Apply leave-in conditioner, then rinse.
- Massage odorless garlic in area where there is loss. Blot; do not rinse.

African

- Mix equal parts of lavender oil, rosemary oil, jojoba oil, jasmine oil, and one part frankincense oil together in a bottle.
- Shampoo, rinse, then massage oil mixture into scalp.
- Use one of the home-conditioning methods—shower steam conditioning, hot towel, or sauna method (explained in detail in Chapter 3, Life in a Bottle) for 15 minutes, then rinse.
- Rosemary should not be used by children under five, pregnant women, or those with high blood pressure, diabetes, or epilepsy.
- Pregnant women should substitute primrose oils for rosemary.

Native American

- Mix equal parts of cedarwood, sage, and sweetgrass/Aveda organics oil.
- Shampoo, then massage oil mixture into scalp. Do not rinse.

Pregnancy

The prefix *bio* comes from the Greek word *bios*, meaning the force of life extended to include organic life. Through pregnancy a woman bears life which is a gift from God. The force of life is manifested through a new human being. While the fetus is growing, hormonal changes are taking place within your body. These changes affect the growth of your hair. The life force increases hair growth. In fact, some women experience tremendous amounts of hair growth. Your texture may even begin to change. However, once your bundle of joy enters into the world, the body goes through trauma and shock that may cause the hair to shed, especially around the hairline. This is known as telogen effluvium. Not to worry. This is only temporary. Your hair will grow back at a normal rate.

TEXTURE MAY CHANGE
DURING PREGNANCY

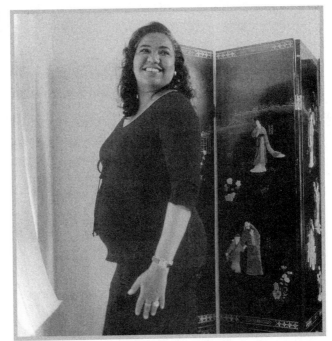

"Telogen effluvium can occur after pregnancy or after trauma to the body such as major surgery, serious illness, or malnutrition," says Dr. Simmons. What can be done? Well, there isn't any pill or medication that is definitely going to make your hair grow back faster. Again, healthy hair grows from the inside out. A proper diet, exercise, and daily supplements are advisable.

Helpful Pregnancy Hints

- Please do not panic, become anxious, or stress about any changes in your hair growth. Relax. Your hair is regenerating itself. Out with the old and in with the new.
- Be patient, which is something you already know about from your pregnancy. I know you want your hair to reflect the joy that has come over you. Instead of stressing, take yoga or Tai Chi classes to help you relax and get your body back into shape.
- Massage a dime-sized amount of shea butter on the scalp and into the shedding areas. This will increase blood circulation and promote hair growth.

I highly recommend staying away from any chemical process while pregnant. Consult with your doctor. Everyone's opinion will be different. Although there aren't any studies on relaxers—only on coloring procedures—applying chemicals during pregnancy may be harmful to the fetus. The choice is ultimately yours. Semipermanent color enhancements are fine for gray coverage or adding hues of color while pregnant.

Many women opt to braid their hair while pregnant, relax their hair less frequently, or simply cut their hair into a short, easy, maintenance-free style while pregnant. Whatever style you choose, you'll always look good. Just remember you're always glowing as you bring a new life force into this world.

Healthy Hair for Children

With children ages 4 to 10, parents should use mild shampoos and conditioners on their tresses. One or two applications of shampoo are sufficient, followed by a leave-in conditioner or instant conditioner. A detangling lotion is advisable when combing the hair after conditioning. And always use a wide-tooth comb for detangling, so your child will feel the least amount of discomfort.

It's always helpful to separate your child's hair into four or five sections with butterfly clips while combing. Detangle each section by holding hair at the base of the scalp and combing from the ends of the hair shaft in a upward direction. Style the hair using plaits, twists, light thermal straightening, blow-drying, and/or roller setting. I recommend Aveda's All Sensitive shampoo and conditioner, Paul Mitchell's

CHILDREN NEED
A TENDER TOUCH

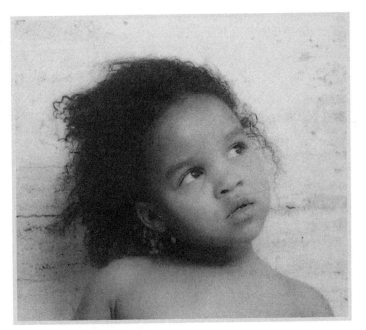

baby shampoo and conditioner, Kiehl's baby shampoo and conditioner, Dr. Bronner's Mild Soap for children, Johnson & Johnson baby shampoo and conditioner, or Aveeno baby wash and shampoo. Ask your doctor for recommendations.

Starting at the age of 9 or 10, young people can begin to use the recommended shampoos in the product section just as you would. At this age you may be considering sending your daughter to a salon for a perm. I suggest staying away from any chemicals until your daughter is ready and able to take full responsibility for the care and maintenance of her tresses. This usually occurs around 15 or 16 years of age. However, I would recommend a texturizer, roller setting, flat ironing, or braids. Consult with your stylist for recommendations.

Scalp & Hair Challenges
Dandruff

Seborrheic dermatitis, commonly known as dandruff, is due to an overgrowth of a type of yeast that lives on the surface of the skin. Dr. Simmons and the dermatological community now understand that the likeliest cause of this overgrowth is an overabundance of oil.

"When a lot of oil is present, the yeast overgrows and breaks up the cells of the top layer of the skin," says Dr. Simmons. "These layers of skin show up as large yellow, greasy scales or flakes." Where do the oils come from? While some people simply produce an overabundance of oil, an increase in oils can also be due to stress or a hormonal imbalance.

"Applying oils and grease to the scalp is a major cultural condition," says Dr. Simmons. "Many women of color have been taught to apply oils and grease to the scalp to control dandruff." This tends to plaster the flakes down and make the condition worse. The type of yeast found in seborrheic dermatitis is an organism normally found on the skin's surface. "We don't know its function. All we can do is try to control it."

According to Dr. Simmons, anecdotally, we can cut back on dairy products and sugar in our diet to help control dandruff. I would also suggest that you go to a nutritionist, who may suggest switching from milk to soy or rice milk and goat cheese. I have personally experienced an overabundance of yeast in my body. Changing my diet was of great help in controlling yeast in my system, on my skin, face, and scalp. I recommend shampooing the scalp with natural anti-inflammatory shampoos such as tea tree, peppermint, or mint shampoos, all of which are discussed in Chapter 3, Life in a Bottle. Most shampoos are fungistatic and slow down the growth of the yeast. In mild cases Dr. Simmons recommends sulfur-, zinc-, or tar-based dandruff shampoos such as Selsun Blue, Original Head & Shoulders, and Neutrogena T/Gel, respectively. She strongly recommends T-Gel for its gentle nature on our hair. Shampoos that are fungicidal actually kill the yeast and they almost always do a better job. Nizoral A-D is one such product. In severe cases, prescription shampoos such as 2% Nizoral shampoo or Lopox shampoo, topical antifungals, steroid lotions, and/or gels are required. New fungicidal agents are expected to be on the market in the near future.

Remember, you should always follow the recommendation of your dermatologist. The stylist and doctor should work in sync to create solutions for scalp conditions and the proper hairstyle. Because these remedies are often very harsh on the hair as well as very drying, I always recommend following the doctor's treatment with a second moisturizing shampoo for the hair shaft.

Psoriasis

Only your dermatologist can diagnose this condition. Thick flakes usually appear on the scalp, accompanied by a great deal of itching. According to Dr. Fran Cook-Bolden, co-author of *Beautiful Skin of Color*, "Psoriasis is seen less frequently in people of color as compared to other diseases involving the scalp." Simple scratching traumatizes the skin, creating an overproduction of cells and causing the skin to flake. Causes of psoriasis may be the environment, genetics, stress, and a compromised immune system. Your dermatologist will select the best treatment depending on the severity. Salicylic acid shampoo helps to break down and remove the flakes and steroids and tar shampoos help with the inflammation. They also work on the overproduction of cell growth. Treatments that contain derivatives of vitamin D work very well, as well as retinoid creams and gels. In severe cases treatment options include injections of steroids, oral medication, and ultraviolet light therapy.

Eczema

Eczema is another condition that should be diagnosed by your doctor. It usually appears as a rash that comes and goes, causing itching of the scalp. It is most often found in families that include one or more persons with allergies, asthma, or hay fever, but not exclusively. You may experience hair loss but it is not permanent. This condition is usually treated with steroid shampoos, tar shampoos, lotions, and gels. Light oils, like canola and hazelnut oils, are essential preparations recommended for psoriasis and eczema and should be used only sparingly on the scalp.

Meditation, a nutritious diet, exercise, a healthy scalp, hair care, and proper maintenance are the key essential ingredients to maintaining healthy hair for those with eczema. Dr. Cook-Bolden also recommends maintaining a good balance of moisture on the scalp by using a light moisturizing cream or lotion.

At-Home Recommendations
- Tea tree shampoos and tea tree oils, which lift flakes and calm inflammation.
- Nizoral shampoo
- Tar-based shampoos

Split Ends
Hair Breakage, Loss, and Shedding

Hair sheds 75 to 100 strands a day. This is normal; however, excessive hair loss may be due to overprocessing of the hair with chemicals, thermal straightening, tight braiding, or pulling the hair back in a ponytail for a long duration. Breakage can also occur when split ends are not caught in time and they ride up the hair shaft, causing breakage. Most times the split ends get caught in your plastic combs and break off. Remember to use a wooden or bone comb to prevent breakage. You can tell where your hair is splitting by running a fine-tooth or wide-tooth comb, depending on your texture, through your hair until the very ends. Wherever the comb stops is usually an indication of where the split end occurs. This is the amount of hair that also should be trimmed off. The other indication is evident: One hair shaft is split in two, hence the term *split ends*.

On a dietary note, split ends can be caused by the excessive consumption of expansive foods like fruit, sugars, raw foods, and salads. Nutritionally, the primary cause of split ends is the excessive consumption of sugars and chemical additives that weaken and starve the hair from the root to tip, according to Christina Pirello. Abusive heat styling is another major factor.

Recommendations include moisturizing the ends of your hair with creams, pomades, laminates, and glosses such as Phytodéfrisant, Phyto 7, Aveda Brilliant pomades, and products containing shea butter. Less frequent use of curling irons and regular trims will prevent split ends, even if you take off only ⅛" every eight weeks. Read more on shaping split ends in Chapter 6, Shear Perfection.

Diet and lifestyle as well as genetics play important roles in whether or not you will suffer hair loss, not to mention the abuse of chemicals and excessive pulling of braids done incorrectly. Eating patterns are passed from generation to generation. A diet and lifestyle change can break the pattern of generations of baldness. Try Phytologie shampoo, conditioner, and vitamins for thin hair.

Baldness has three basic causes and occurs in certain patterns. When there is an increase of testosterone or androgen (male hormones), you may experience hair loss. This is the reason men bald, according to Dr. Simmons. Consequently, women bald when there isn't enough estrogen or female hormones to combat the androgen hormone.

"There is a school of thought that believes that testosterone levels play a large part in hair growth," says Dr. Simmons. "We experience seasonal hair growth (summer, fall, winter, and spring) just like animals. T-levels, if you will, peak in the fall when we see the most hair loss and are lowest in the spring. Therefore, spring is when hair grows the most. Some studies held with large groups of women have shown these exact results."

High testosterone levels may cause alopecia or male pattern baldness, typically baldness in the center of the head. However, the same type of balding can also be seen when testosterone levels are normal. We cannot fully explain this. According to nutritionist Christina Pirello, hair can drop off when there is too much saturated fat in the body. An increase in animal protein in our diet may cause thinning hair in women as well as men. Controlling your blood sugar levels and balancing your diet can help you regulate your testosterone levels, therefore increasing or decreasing hair growth. Ask your dermatologist for more information. Remember, if you never ask, you'll never know.

Dermatologist Dr. Fran Cook-Bolden suggests treating this type of alopecia with minoxidil, a prescribed treatment. The shampoos, conditioners, and topical solutions are also sold under the brand name Rogaine. Interestingly enough, minoxidil was first used for high blood pressure, and a side effect was hair growth. Now researched and tested to treat hair loss, it is sold at drug stores and in salons. You may see wonderful results with minoxidil but if you stop using it you may experience hair loss again. Please follow your doctor's instructions carefully.

Alopecia is the general term for hair loss. One of the most common forms of alopecia seen by hairstylists is alopecia areata. It may appear as a dime-, nickel- or quarter-sized area on the scalp where the skin is smooth and shiny and no hair is present. The condition is usually spotted by your stylist, who may suggest you see a dermatologist. It may develop rather suddenly and is caused by a minor defect in the immune system. Medical treatment by your dermatologist often involves use of corticosteroids. This type of alopecia can be associated with thyroid disease and diabetes, but is most often due to severe stress.

Alopecia seborrheica is hair loss caused by severe cases of seborrheic dermatitis. Once the yeast is under control, your hair will begin to grow back normally.

Traction alopecia occurs when there is trauma to the hair follicle, causing thinning along the sides of the temples. This is the most common form of alopecia seen by hairstylists. Usually this occurs when braids are placed too tightly or the hair is pulled back in a ponytail too tightly for an extended period of time. It can also be seen in any area of the scalp if the hair is pulled too tightly, e.g., with tight rollers. Dr. Cook-Bolden has found this type of alopecia to be extremely difficult to treat if treatment is delayed. So, it is important to seek treatment immediately for best results. According to nutritionist Christina Pirello, traction alopecia is caused by pulling tightly on the hair combined with an excessive intake of fruit juices and acidic soft drinks.

However, I have found that if traction alopecia is caught early and the follicle has not been destroyed (as diagnosed by a dermatologist), applying and massaging shea butter to the area three to four times a week for one month will result in some hair growth.

I firmly recommend that you ask your stylist not to braid your hair very tightly. Let her know that you would rather come in for regular touch-ups than have your hair braided tightly. I always recommend that braids be washed and steam-conditioned every two to three weeks, with touch-ups on the braids at every visit.

If the stylist doesn't comply, then stop going to that person. Yes, I said STOP. It's not worth it. Headaches are unacceptable and so is pulling your hair back. If you constantly pull your hair back and it is falling out, I suggest you skip right to Chapter 6, Shear Perfection, for advice on choosing a new style.

Androgenetic alopecia occurs during the perimenopausal and menopausal states. It may be caused by elevated levels of testosterone in the hair follicles. Women may not have enough estrogen to counteract the androgen hormone during this time in their lives.

"When this occurs in young women, often it represents an abnormal hormonal state," says Dr. Simmons. With polycystic ovarian syndrome, women may experience irregular periods, acne, and hair loss. This is just helpful information. Please do not become alarmed if you are experiencing any of these symptoms. Simply go to your doctor. Often your doctor can determine your condition right away.

Repeated trauma to the follicle caused by rollers, combing hair too harshly, and constant use of curling irons are common causes of follicular degeneration syndrome (FDS) or central centrifugal alopecia (CCA). Very common among black women, this type of hair loss starts at the crown of the head and slowly expands. The scalp appears shiny and slightly scarred. According to Dr. Simmons, in previous years the main cause was thought to be hot combing. However, it is still being seen today even though natural styling has become more prevalent. Steroid injections may be prescribed. In severe cases hair transplants are recommended. Other than these treatments, it is important for ladies not to overuse tools and abuse your hair. Following the proper direction and guidance suggested in Chapter 4, Diane's Bag, will assist you tremendously.

According to Christina Pirello, edibles such as whole grains, fermented foods, and pickles feed the blood with nutrients. Blood feeds the pulpi, which in turn feed the hair follicles, increasing hair growth and reducing hair loss. When cholesterol levels in the blood are normal, blood circulates freely, with no blockages, feeding the hair efficiently and thoroughly. Foods that are rich in living enzymes, such as soybeans, ease the digestive system and fortify the quality of the blood, nourishing the body and hair with essential oils, vitamins, and minerals.

In addition to fermented foods and pickles, soy sauce, tamari, and miso are also very good for the hair, miso being the most beneficial. Miso is made from soybeans, whole grain, and salt and is rich in living enzymes.

Sea plants are also important for maintenance of our hair's health. Rich in beta-carotene, sea plants help prevent the buildup of dead skin cells that can clog the hair follicles, inhibiting the growth and health of the hair. B vitamins are also linked to the prevention of oily hair, baldness, and dandruff. Calcium is essential to the structure of the hair shaft. Phosphorous, potassium, sulphur, magnesium, and copper aid in giving color to the hair. Selenium bromine and other sea plants are key foods for preventing premature gray hair.

Hair loss can also be attributed to stress. Stress can come from outside influences of daily living. And of course, there are various stress levels. Signs of stress are stomachaches, headaches, nervous energy, worry, and anxiety, which can all lead to hair loss and hair shedding. Constant nervous twisting of the hair causes the hair to fall out from the roots.

Stress management is a positive technique for controlling and preventing stress, which in turn will reduce hair loss. Dr. Henry McCurtis, head of psychiatric medicine at Harlem Hospital and in private practice in New York City, suggests combining a three-part stress management technique that is spiritually, physically, and mentally based.

Physically

Fifteen minutes of aerobics in the morning prompts the heart to generate a flow of blood that circulates to the brain and scalp, which feeds the follicles and promotes hair growth.

Mentally

Try this meditating and breathing technique: breathe in, hold your breath and count for 10 to 15 seconds, and then release while envisioning a beautiful peaceful environment such as the ocean or the lush greenery of mountains. This promotes a calm and tranquil disposition. Positive thoughts prepare you to take on environmental stresses during the day.

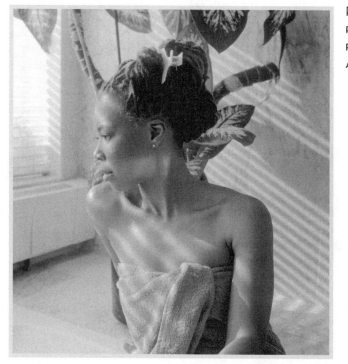

RELAX AND RELEASE STRESS FROM YOUR HAIR AND YOUR LIFE

Spiritually

Praising the Father, giving thanks, and counting all your blessings acknowledges that all is right with the world. Believing that the Creator has you in the palm of His hands reduces worry and internal stress, which in turn can control nervousness, including hair loss from pulling and tugging out your hair. Knowing and living by faith promotes peace and order.

I personally combine aerobics, yoga, meditation, and prayer as my daily routine each and every morning. I drink an herbal protein drink, Namaska's Muntu Green Drink, mixed with my favorite juices, and take my vitamins and supplements. For my daily spiritual enforcement throughout the day, I read my Bible, create and adhere to positive thinking, stay away from petty gossip, and surround myself with positive people.

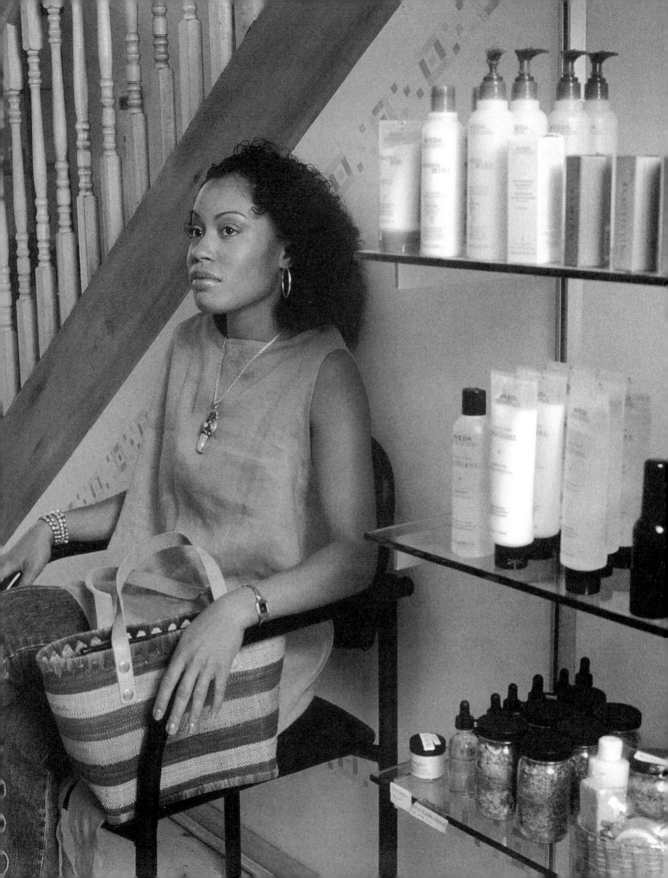

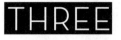

THREE

Life in a Bottle
Products to Maintain Your Tresses

I always seek out and experiment with the right products that work for my hair texture.

—Kym Christensen, fashion designer

Healthy Hair

There are four different hair types: oily, normal, dry, and damaged (overprocessed). Always select the right shampoo for your specific hair type. You should wash your hair at least once a week. Though it may not seem like it, I assure you that it is a myth that dirty hair is more manageable. My rule of thumb is if you have to scratch your scalp more than once, that's one time too many. Your scalp must be cleaned and your hair should always be shampooed. Shampooing once a week keeps the hair free of debris and provides a pathway for natural oils to lubricate the scalp and hair. Short natural hair (from Caesar length to two inches of hair), can be shampooed every day or every other day. After shampooing, apply a leave-in conditioner. For those who work out consistently, you should shampoo every three to four days or when necessary.

It is essential to know how to properly shampoo your hair in order to have a healthy scalp. The first thing you should do is a water wash, which is rinsing the hair with tepid water for two to three minutes to

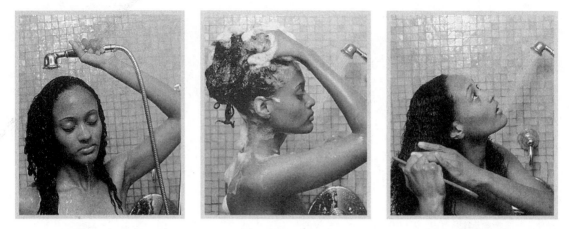

WATER WASH | SHAMPOO | COMBING THROUGH CONDITIONER

lift and loosen any debris and buildup of gels and products. The first shampoo is the cleansing shampoo and is rather minimal. Your second shampoo should lather more abundantly. Massage with fingertips as you shampoo the crown of the head and work your hands to the hairline and nape of the neck.

Conditioners should be applied every time you shampoo your hair. Remember, conditioning can do only so much for hair repair. It can mend and coat the hair shaft; however, if the hair is completely damaged, has split ends, and/or is shedding, the only alternative may be to have the damaged hair cut by a professional. We'll discuss more about the importance of keeping textured hair shaped regularly in Chapter 6, Shear Perfection. Starting over with a healthy head of hair is always the better solution. I know you don't want to hear it because sisters especially like to hold on to their hair. I can't stress enough the importance of following a healthy maintenance plan.

If your hair is tightly coiled, you can even leave a little conditioner in the hair when you're rinsing it for more manageability. Leave-in conditioners can be applied before applying gel on wavy or frizzy hair.

Steam conditioning invigorates the scalp. Conditioner and/or herbal

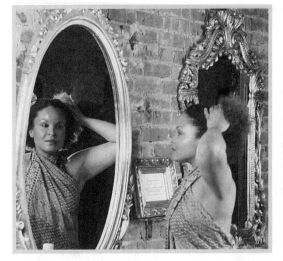

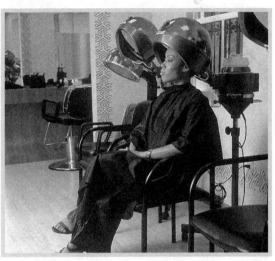

APPLYING LEAVE-IN CONDITIONER

STEAMING ALLOWS CONDITIONER TO
PENETRATE THE HAIR SHAFT

oil is massaged into the scalp before the head is placed under a steamer. The water vapors open the outer layer of the hair shaft with moisture, allowing the conditioner to penetrate deeply into the cuticle layer. Steam conditioning promotes hair growth, which is why the steamer is an essential treatment. At my salon, botanical and herbal treatments are applied to the scalp and massaged in. However, I also use a deep conditioner/essential oil mixture, which also happens to be an Asian crème bath treatment. Afterward, the client is placed under the steamer for about 15 to 20 minutes. This is especially good for locs, natural hair, and color-treated hair.

There are many ways to steam your hair outside of the salon setting. However, steaming at home is only meant to hold you over until you can get an appointment with your professional stylist. The home treatment is helpful to your at-home maintenance when you are unable to get to the salon. However, there is absolutely no substitute for a professional steam treatment.

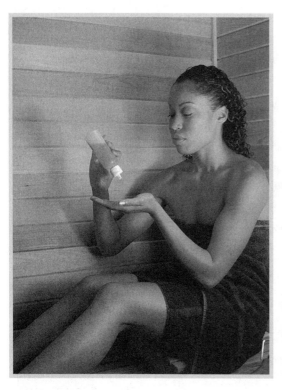

POURING HERBAL OILS

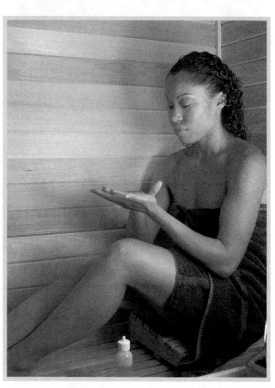

RUBBING OILS IN PALMS

After you've massaged the oils and/or deep conditioner into your hair, you can place a hot towel over your head for 15 minutes. You can also sit in a steam sauna or create your own sauna by running hot water in the shower for 15 minutes and filling the bathroom with steam.

Deep-penetrating and reconstructing conditioners should be applied and then combed through the hair before placing the head under a heating cap, or sitting under a hair dryer with a plastic cap for 15 to 20 minutes. Afterward, your hair should be rinsed and combed out.

Stay away from products containing mineral oil, petrolatum, and

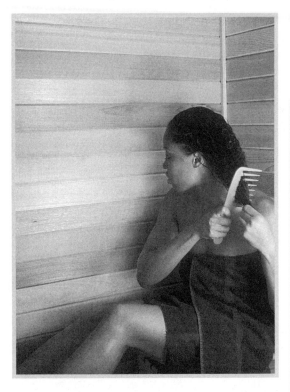

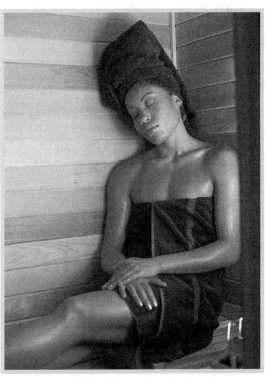

NOW, RELAX

beeswax. They will create a heavy film on the hair. Also, wax tends to weigh your hair down and attract a great deal of dirt and debris. When applying a protein conditioner to overstressed or processed hair, be certain to follow up with a light cream or leave-in conditioner to soften the hair. Pure protein tends to harden the hair.

Now that we're on the right path to healthy, happy hair, it's important for us to choose the right weaponry—that is, the right shampoos, conditioners, and finishing products—and it's just as significant to know when to use them. So let's begin by differentiating among the various types of shampoos.

Clarifying and cleansing shampoos lift debris and environmental pollutants from the hair. I recommend Aveda Rosemary Mint shampoo, Aveda Detoxifier shampoo, Paul Mitchell Tea Tree Special Shampoo, Kiehl's Peppermint shampoo, and Carol's Daughter Rosemary Mint shampoo.

Moisturizing shampoos contain humectants that attract moisture. Some of my favorites are Kiehl's, Origins, Aveda Sap Moss, Dove, Mizani, Graham Webb, Phytospecific Vitaforce shampoo with macadamia oil, Phyto Mousse, and Neutrogena.

Conditioning shampoos are used to treat dry, brittle, and damaged hair as well as chemically treated and color processed hair. I've successfully worked with Aveda Shampure, Aveda Curessence, Goldwell Definition Shampoo, PhytoRhum, Mizani, Kiehl's, and Pantene Pro-V for relaxed and natural hair.

Dandruff and medicated shampoos treat the scalp and are not really formulated to treat the hair. They are medicated with natural ingredients such as tea tree oil, zinc, or tar, which slow down the cell growth and discourage fungal infections. However, they can be very harsh on the hair. I recommend Paul Mitchell Tea Tree Special Shampoo, Kera-Care Dry and Itchy Scalp shampoo, and Natural Uplift Root Stimulator. Over-the-counter tar- or zinc-based shampoos such as Nizoral are very effective as well. I always suggest to my clients that they begin with a tepid water wash, then massage in a dime- to quarter-sized amount of dandruff or medicated shampoo, depending on the thickness of the hair. It's important to follow up with a moisturizing or conditioning shampoo to treat the hair shaft.

Hair cannot live by shampoo alone, so always follow a thorough shampoo with good conditioning. Here are the different types:

Instant conditioners are applied and left in the hair for five minutes, combed through, and rinsed out. They can be used as a regular part of your shampoo/conditioner regimen.

Leave-in conditioners are self-explanatory. They're simply conditioners left in the hair without rinsing out. Apply conditioner, comb through with a wide-tooth comb, then style as usual. Aveda Elixir, PhytoLightbalm, Goldwell leave-in-conditioner spray, and Graham Webb Synchronicity are all very good. Synchronicity is very concentrated, so use it sparingly. It also works well as a deep conditioner.

Deep penetrating or restructuring conditioners should be used once a month or every two weeks depending on the condition of the hair, especially after braids are removed. These conditioners are applied to the hair and combed through with a wide-tooth comb, then the hair is placed under a heating cap or plastic cap under a hair dryer for 15 to 20 minutes. Afterward, rinse out the conditioner and comb through. Try Goldwell Definition Color & Highlights Treatment, Kerasilk, Aveda Curessence, PhytoMoelle, Phytospecific Cream Bath, or L'Oréal Kérastase Conditioner.

Botancial and herbal treatments are best done at the salon. The conditioning oil is applied to the scalp, massaged in, and then the client is placed under a steamer. I've been doing this treatment for over 10 years and highly recommend it, especially for locked, natural, and color-treated hair. I've also used a treatment consisting of a deep conditioner and an essential oil mixed together in a bowl, then applied to the client's hair shaft. The client is placed under the steamer for 15 to 20 minutes. This is also known as an Asian crème bath treatment. I really like Aveda Energizing Nutrients, Phyto Huile D'Ales, Lisa's Hair Elixir, and Mizani Moisture Comfort Oil as herbal oil treatments. All these treatments can be achieved at home using the hot towel, sauna, or hot steam method.

Moisturizing conditioners attract moisture to the hair. KeraCare Humecto, Aveda Brilliant Conditioner, Aveda Sap Moss, Dove, Mizani Moisture Fuse, Neutrogena, and Pantene Pro-V are great ones.

Color conditioners maintain the vibrancy of your hair color between visits to the salon and should be used after every washing. Try Biolage Earth Tones Color Reserve and Aveda Color Conserve conditioners.

Shea butter is a conditioner, moisturizer, and healing agent for the scalp. It is made from the West African shea nut. It's also a great skin moisturizer and is excellent for controlling hair loss. I first used shea butter while working at Kinapps. I'd advise clients who'd experienced hair loss from braiding and stress to massage the shea butter into their scalp every night for three weeks. They always came back with new hair growth, as long as the hair follicle in the area had not been completely damaged. You can also use a small amount of shea butter on the ends of the hair to prevent them from splitting or riding up the hair shaft. Pure shea butter is very heavy, so always use it sparingly. Try Frédéric Fekkai or Carol's Daughter shea butter products.

Essential oils include rosemary, lavender, sage, and ylang-ylang. Read Chapter 2, Healthy Hair Is Happy Hair, for a more extensive list.

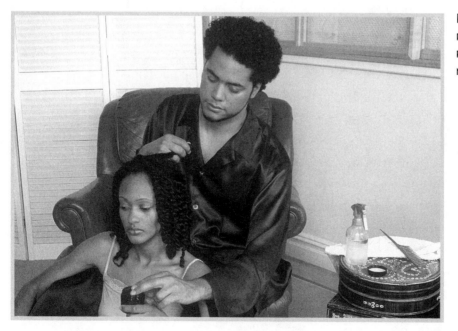

EXPERIMENT WITH PRODUCTS AND FIND THE PERFECT MATCH FOR YOU

Though I've experimented with all kinds of products throughout my career, I only use products that have botanical ingredients and plant and flower essences. You'll notice the difference in your hair in just two to three washings after switching over from synthetic-based products.

Finishing products are glosses and sheens, pomades, herbal and essential oils, gels, waxes, mousse, hair spray, and molding and sculpturing pomades and waxes. Because we'll use these sparingly and only after the hair is styled, I'll explain their uses and recommend specific brands in Part 2, Achieve It! Styling Your Textured Hair.

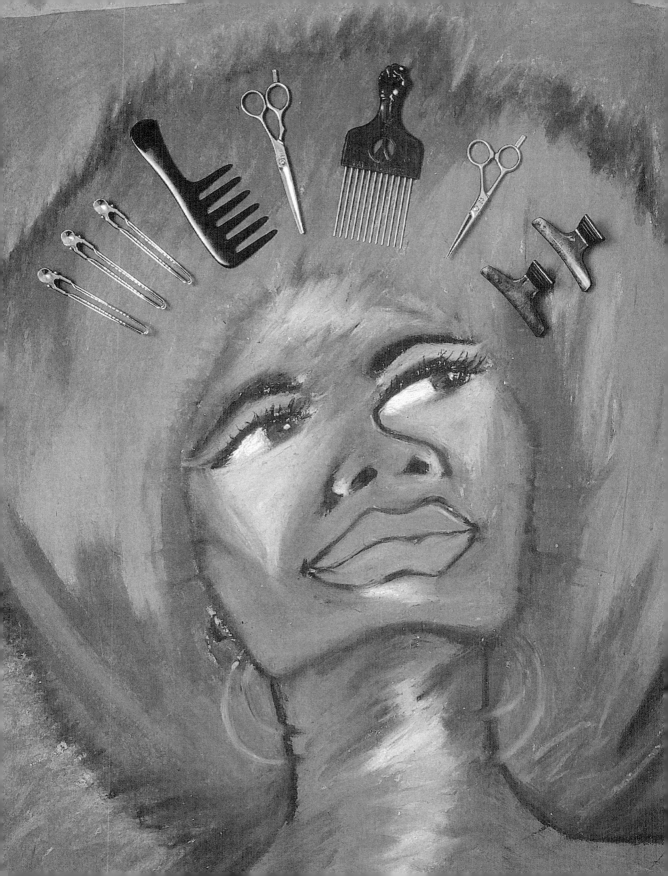

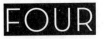

Diane's Bag

Tools You Need for Proper Hair Care

Order and the organization of your tools are the keys to successful styling. —Diane Da Costa

hink about it. What would a painter be without her brush? A chef without a spatula? A doctor without a stethoscope? You get the idea, ladies. The right tools are essential to healthy hair care and proper styling. I carry my Cynthia Rowley bag with me on my personal visits to service my clients. What's in my bag? All of my light equipment such as combs, brushes, blow-dryers, and products. However, when I have to carry everything but the kitchen sink, I have a neat, organized, professional styling pulley that has separate compartments for all my tools like flatirons, curling irons, rollers, you name it. I also carry a leather rollup case designed by Denise Kerr to store my combs, shears, and clips.

I like all my tools and products to be very organized. The leather case pictured here is perfect for me. I just stick all my tools right in their specially designed sections, roll it up, and go. If not, I'll hastily throw everything in a bag in a rush, resulting in disorder. I'm very meticulous and a perfectionist, so I try to stay away from chaos and confusion. God likes order, and where there is confusion there are other negative elements. Organize your tools, brushes, clips, and accessories. My client

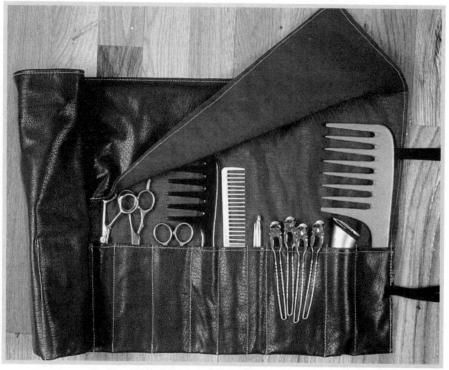

Kym Christensen, a fashion and home interior designer, suggests putting them in separate baskets.

I clean all of my tools after every use. However, if you're the only one using your tools, you should wash them once a week with liquid sanitizer, like Sea Breeze, or do Barbicide like the salons. Also, wipe your electronic styling tools with a damp cloth after every use to prevent product buildup.

With that said, continuing on the path of order and organization, here are the tools I love to use on all my clients.

Combs

I personally use **bone combs** by Pivot Point for basic combing.

Large fantail combs are used for detangling wavy, curly, and very curly hair that is longer than five inches.

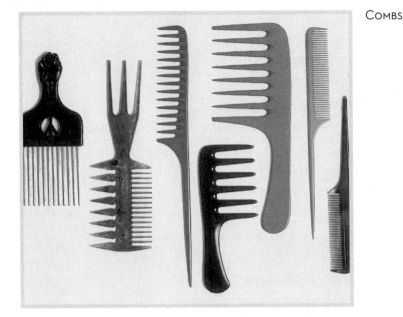

Small fantail combs are used for precise parting and applying chemical relaxers.

Large wide-tooth combs with handles are used to separate and detangle damp and wet hair after applying conditioner or detangling lotion.

Large wide-tooth combs are used for parting and combing through detangled hair.

Metal picks are normally used to pick out afros or to loosen hair completely before trimming. They can also be used to style various looks like the Twist Out for extra lift.

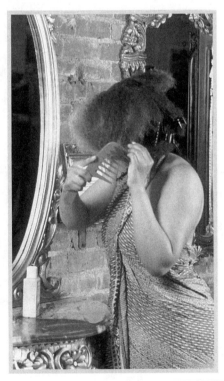

A WIDE-TOOTH COMB IS A MUST-HAVE FOR VERY CURLY HAIR

Styling combs are used for lifting, separating, styling, defining, and sculpturing all textures.

Tortoiseshell claws and tortoiseshell picks and combs are used for both styling and lifting.

Small black wide-tooth combs are used for basic combing.

Brushes

Wide paddle brushes are used for blow-drying, wrapping the hair, and massaging the scalp.

Oval boar bristle brushes are used to blow-dry straight and wavy hair. They can also be used to brush hair at night or for wrapping dry hair. Men can also use oval boar bristle brushes for overall brushing and for placement.

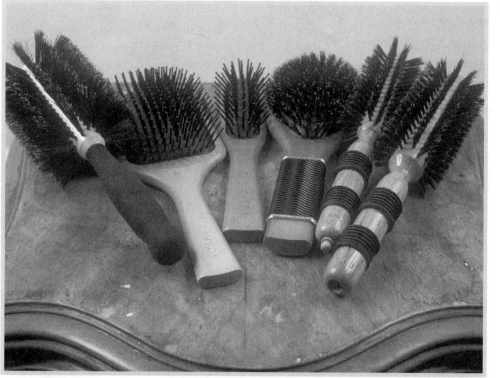

BRUSHES

Round brushes (small, medium, and large) are used for blow-drying. I recommend blow-drying with the **Denman Brush** for a smooth shiny finish on texturized and relaxed hair.

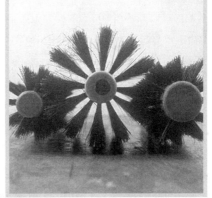

Shears

Shears should be left in the hands of the professionals. I do not recommend that you cut, trim, or shape your own hair. Nonetheless, I do think it is important for you to know and understand what tools professionals use on your head.

I use 5" and 5½" shears for precision cutting and 6" shears for overall shaping. Shears can also be used for chopping and slicing the hair to give it a jagged and multidimensional shape.

Texturizing shears are shears with wide teeth or a comb-like blade on one side and a solid blade on the other side. I use texturizing shears for softening relaxed hair, removing bulk from wavy hair, and creating a wispy look around the face and edges. Texturizing the hair with shears adds dimension and a natural flow and movement. I often texturize a cut into the edges of the hair to create shape while keeping length.

SHEARS

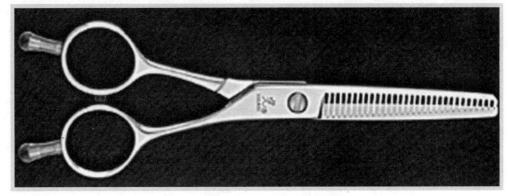

Razors

Razors are used to create definition and for blending. Blending and slicing are two popular methods.

Blow-Dryers

I don't recommend ever blow-drying the hair with an attachment as your first heat application. It will dry out the hair, create unwanted split ends, and pull damaged hair right out of your head. Please don't abuse your hair with the overuse of blow-dryers. Use the blow-dryer sparingly, air drying the hair when possible.

Instead of using an attachment, I recommend using a blow-dryer and paddle brush for wavy and curly hair; a blow-dryer and a round brush for straight, wavy, and relaxed hair; and a blow-dryer and large-tooth comb for very curly and tightly coiled hair until hair is semi-straight on medium heat. Follow with blow-dryer and comb attachment on medium heat.

I use the Elchim Baby Bliss Ionic, Solis, and Super Solano 1250-watt

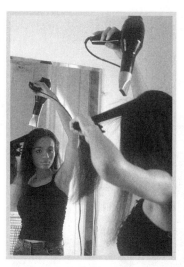

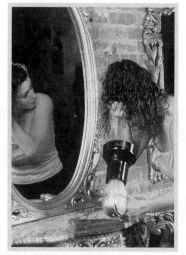

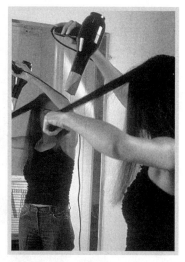

BLOW-DRYER SHOULD BE AT LEAST TWELVE INCHES FROM THE HAIR

USE A DIFFUSER ATTACHMENT TO DEFINE YOUR CURL PATTERN

BLOW-DRYER SHOULD FOLLOW THE MOVEMENT OF THE BRUSH

blow-dryers. Medium heat is generally warm enough to dry hair of any texture. All textures can air dry or be placed under a hooded dryer on medium heat to remove excess water before blow-drying. Generally speaking, very curly and tightly coiled hair that is relaxed should be dried under a hooded dryer for a few minutes prior to blow-drying; however, straight and wavy hair tends to achieve a better finish when blow-dried wet or damp. The less heat applied to the hair, the better the long-term results. So ladies, please try to keep the stress and pressure on your hair to a minimum. Apply leave-in conditioner and gel before using a diffuser (an attachment to the blow-dryer that minimizes air pressure and dries the hair in place).

Flat Irons

After the hair has been blown dry, flat irons can be used to straighten all textures for a smooth, silky, straight look.

The model Jessica separates the hair into sections panel by panel with a bone comb. Then she places the flat iron on the hair ½ inch away from the scalp, sliding both the comb and iron down the shaft until straight.

I recommend the Kenya flat iron and the Baby Bliss flat iron.

FLAT IRONS GIVE YOU A
SMOOTH, SILKY FINISH

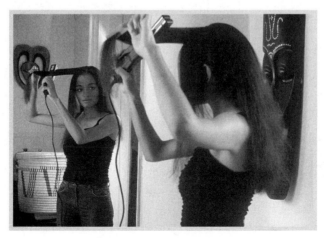

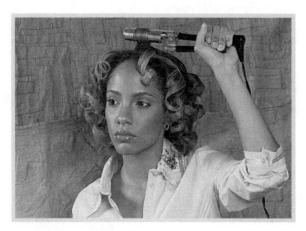

Curling Irons

Electric barrel curling irons create different sized curls using electric heat. They're great for wavy, curly, or relaxed hair. Very curly and tightly coiled hair generally retain heat when curled with a Marcel Barrel Curling Iron or Kizuri curling irons. Usually these irons are what you'll find your stylist using, and again, they should be left in the hands of a professional. (See Chapter 8, Natural Sets and Styles.)

Again, please don't abuse your hair with irons. After curling or flat ironing, try wrapping the hair or pin curling by creating a large curl and securing it with a pin.

Clips

Butterfly clips are used to hold large sections of already separated textured hair as well as locs.

Ducktail and large silver clips hold separated locs while palm rolling or retightening new growth. These clips are also used to hold separated straight, relaxed, and blow-dried textured hair while curling or flat-ironing.

Hairpins

Large and small hairpins are used for styling all textures.

Elastic Bands

Stay away from rubber bands. Use elastic cloth bands or scrunchies instead.

I also carry certain products in my bag along with my tools. These are the jars and bottles I like to keep with me:

Carol's Daughter Mimosa Hair Honey

Aveda Brilliant Hair Spray

Aveda Brilliant Humectant Pomade

Aveda Light Elements Shine

Graham Webb Styling Mousse

Graham Webb Wax Pomade

My custom-blended mixture of sesame, lavender, rosemary, jasmine, and frankincense oils

I'll instruct you further on the proper use of all these tools in Part 2, Achieve It! Styling Your Textured Hair.

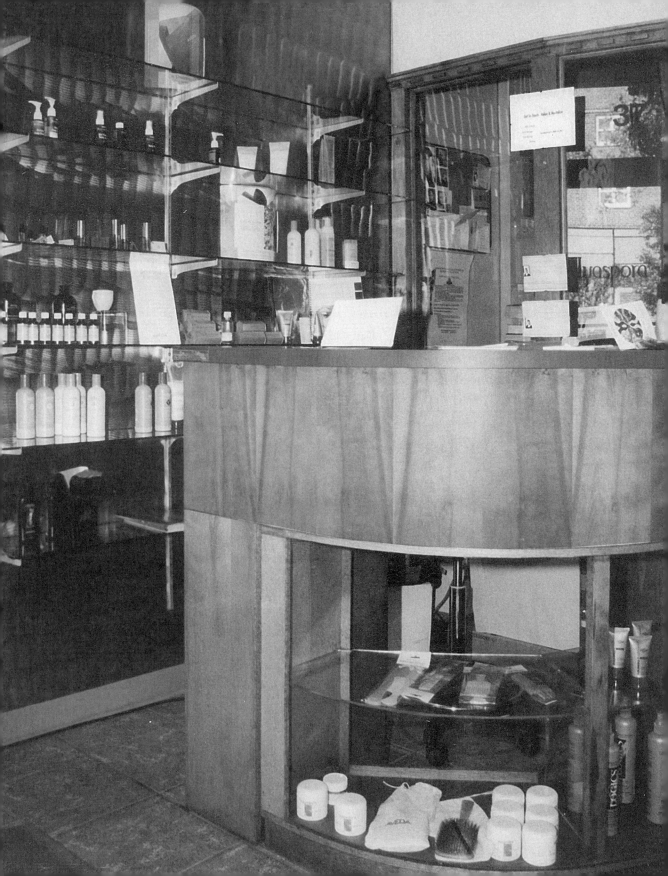

FIVE

In Harmony
Picking the Right Stylist and Salon

Peace is good karma. —Diane Da Costa

By the time you're done reading this book, you'll probably think you can take care of your beautifully textured hair all by yourself. Perhaps you even thought that way before you ever picked up this book. Or maybe that very thought is the reason you grabbed the book off the shelf or added it to your shopping cart online in the first place. Dare I dig deeper and say that not wanting to bother with a salon or a stylist is the main reason you wear your hair natural or are thinking of going natural? Well, I'm here to break that train of thinking right here and right now. Natural hair, textured hair, does not always equate to wash-and-wear hair. Ladies, there are just some things—like cutting, coloring, texturizing, and, let's face it, certain styling—that are best left in the hands of a trusted professional.

Already open to the idea of a hair professional working on your head? Great. Then maybe you are the type of client who stays loyal to her hair stylist for years and years or the trendy client who jumps around from salon to salon because she must be serviced at the "hot" salon of the moment. Regardless of who you are and what you're working with, it's important to choose the right hair professional, the right hair partner, if

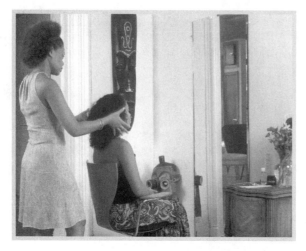

you will, to assist you in your effort of growing, maintaining, and styling your textured hair.

First and most important, a thorough consultation is essential to connecting with the right hair partner. Observe the stylist's overall ability and skills. Maybe you've seen his or her work in a magazine or on the head of the well-coiffed person sitting next to you on the train or sitting at a stoplight. Get their name and number and schedule a consultation with the stylist at the salon. Most salons offer a 10- to 15-minute consultation at no charge. Once you've scheduled your consultation, you may want to bring along a few pictures to give the stylist an idea of the style you have in mind for yourself.

On the day of your appointment, feel free to ask about his or her training and advanced education. Ask whether the style is high- or low-maintenance. Inquire about at-home care and follow-up visits. Don't be afraid to ask about the costs. No one knows your budget better than you. Open communication and clarity between the stylist and client are crucial.

The stylist should definitely be concerned about the healthiness of your hair. In fact, here's a list of a few things that should happen on the day of your appointment.

1. Expect to be greeted in a friendly and cordial manner.

2. Expect to be faced toward the mirror and conversed with openly about your past hair history.

3. Expect to be asked about chemicals (if any) and products used on your hair.

4. Expect to be given an elasticity/porosity test. Stylist should comb through hair and observe both the elasticity and porosity of your hair.

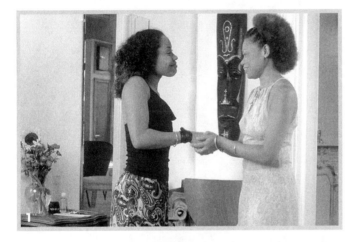

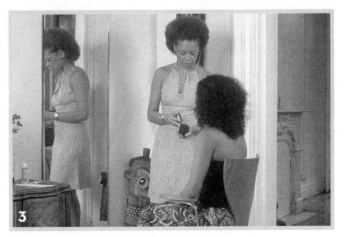

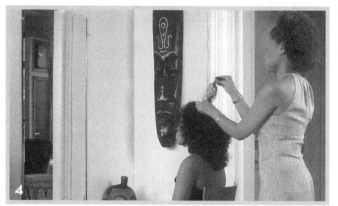

ELASTICITY

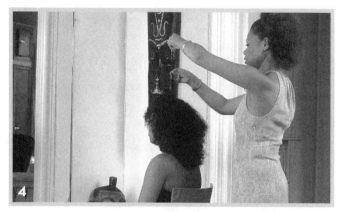

POROSITY

5. Expect to be asked about your lifestyle, be it active or sedentary.

6. Expect to be told the truth about the style you have in mind. If the stylist feels that it is not the right style for you, he or she should definitely offer you alternatives and solutions.

7. Expect to be informed about the procedure, technique, and the time involved.

8. Expect to be told the price. The stylist should tell you whether the services are all inclusive or à la carte.

9. Expect to listen to your gut instinct as to whether this person is indeed the right partner for you. Whom you choose to help you care, maintain, and style your hair is a sacred choice.

Once you've found the right partner, it's important that the two of you establish a good hair program. I always prescribe for my clients strict instruction on maintenance and at-home care, and routine visits and products.

I love change. I especially love changing hair color seasonally. All change is good as long as the hair is kept healthy. I also like progress. Once I get you on the healthy hair program, that's where I want you to stay. My clients can't always find me when they need me, so they know how to take care of their hair in the meantime; if that doesn't work, then I'm more than happy to refer them to someone else if they so choose.

A client usually stays with a particular stylist for around seven years. After that many feel like they need a change. So off they go to another hair stylist. They often find their way back to me with all types of hair stories, and I never get offended. Why? Because that's how the universe works. The universe provides new clients to replace the old ones and when the old clients come back they appreciate me even more. It is a life lesson.

Stylists are human. You can outgrow your stylist and want a change. But please remember, it is so much better to part with friendship and recommendations than to leave gossiping and in anger.

Now that you have a good sense of what to look for in a good hair partner, take a glance at the hair professional glossary below to assist you in knowing what or who you are looking for. Keep in mind we are talking about licensed, experienced, and skilled hair care specialists here.

Hair Stylist: one who may have vision in his/her own right and can also duplicate popular styles.

Hair Designer: an artist who creates the trends in hair. Hair designers are inspired by art and life and are able to create their vision, the style, from the canvas, which is your hair.

Hair Care Specialist: one who knows how to determine the healthiness of the hair through proper analysis and then cares for the hair through products, treatments, and shaping. Ideally you should find a hair care specialist and a designer. They are rarely one and the same.

Natural Hair Care Specialist: the same as above, but he or she specializes in natural hairstyles as well as the care of natural hair using products with botanical ingredients.

Colorist: a hair professional who has been trained and is certified by a color company, and has received continuing education courses from manufacturers and recognizes seasonal trends. Many hair stylists can apply color, but not every hair stylist is a colorist. A colorist has a keen eye for choosing, formulating, creating, and blending colors.

Master Precision Cutter: one who is able to shape and cut all texture, whether it is naturally or chemically straight, wavy, curly, very curly, or tightly coiled. Precision cutters have trained with some of the best cutting academies in the United States and/or abroad.

Master Braider: one who has mastered all the techniques of braided styles.

Loctician: one who specializes in the care, maintenance, grooming, and styling of locs.

Smart clients always have at least two stylists they can count on. It may work for you to have different professionals to serve different needs—one to help you care for your hair (hair care specialist/natural hair care specialist), another to cut your hair (precision cutter), a colorist, and a braider. It's very rare that you find a stylist who does everything. However, when looking for a stylist, consider the hair care specialist for your main stylist. At the very least your stylist should be able to care for your hair, cut and style. Seek out experienced professionals when you want the other added benefits like coloring and braiding.

While I recognize local braid shops, "suga shops," and salons for quick blow-drying in many of our communities, I cannot with good conscience recommend them all. Often people go to them because they're cheaper than natural hair salons, but as the adage goes, "you get what you pay for." At a natural hair salon you're paying for actual hair care (i.e., shampoo, conditioner, and advice on touch-ups), while many local braid shops don't even have sinks in them. You're also paying for high-quality styling, twisting, and braiding. After visiting local braid shops, many new clients have complained of experiencing pain during the braiding process and hair loss due to traction alopecia. At a reputable natural salon you will be surrounded by cleanliness and comfort.

WHAT TO LOOK FOR IN A SALON

1. Clean environment

2. Well designed and organized

3. No clutter

4. Helpful customer service

5. One or two product lines available for use and for sale

6. Team work

7. No gossiping

While I've provided you with information on how to care for your hair in the previous chapters, keep in mind that certified stylists and salons are available to assist you in your mission for achieving healthy, happy textured hair. It's like childbirth—you can deliver a baby all by yourself; women have been doing it for centuries. But isn't it comforting to know to know there are qualified midwives and obstetricians at your service should you need them? Think about it.

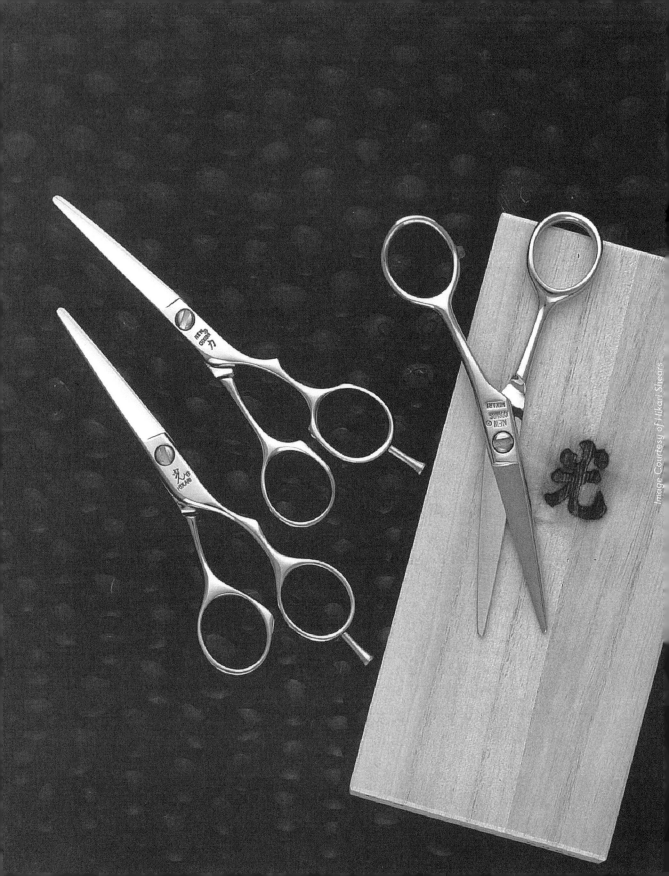

SIX

Shear Perfection

The Necessity for Change via Shaping and Cutting

My hair is like a snake's skin. I must shed it every six months. There's so much energy in my hair after I travel to Europe for the fashion shows. I have to get it out. Just cut it. Just cut it. Just cut it!

—Pamela Macklin, fashion editor, *Essence* magazine

"Remember, I just want a trim, not a cut!" Does this sound like you? Admit it—some of you ladies actually flinch when your stylist picks up her shears to trim or cut your hair. Perhaps it's the fear of the unknown that makes you so nervous. Well, fear no more. I want you to have a better understanding, a working knowledge of cutting and trimming. Once you have that, I believe all of the trauma associated with cutting and trimming will be history, or at least lessened. By no means am I suggesting you cut your own hair. This chapter is meant to serve as a guideline for what you should expect from your stylist. By the way, trimming, cutting, shaping, it's all the same to me. As long as I have to pick up my shears, I always see this as cutting your hair. The only difference is the amount of inches you want taken off as opposed to a complete change with a style cut.

According to precision cutter Felipe, the basic cutting principles are the same for textured hair as they are for straight, wavy, or curly hair.

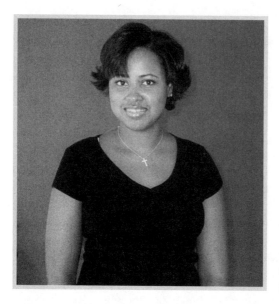

A GREAT CUT IS THE FOUNDATION FOR ALL TEXTURES

"There is a particular format that we need to follow," says Felipe, "starting with the bone and facial structure, facial proportions, and the whole cranial structure in its entirety. That's what we need to understand. These are the basic principles we need to know and understand to cut basically any type of hair."

Whether your hair is naturally textured, texturized, or relaxed, it's always important to have your hair shaped. *Shaping* is the new buzzword, rather than *trimming* or *cutting*, though really it's all the same. I recommend shaping every two months for naturally textured hair, particularly to keep your ends from splitting and riding up the hair shaft.

For texturized and relaxed hair I recommend getting your hair shaped approximately every six to eight weeks, usually around the time you're having your chemical process applied. There have been several books suggesting that you don't have to shape your ends while you're growing your hair longer. I agree with this as long as you don't abuse your hair with tools such as blow-dryers and curling irons, and as long as you keep your ends moisturized with laminates, glosses, or moisturizers such as shea butter to prevent split ends while you're growing your

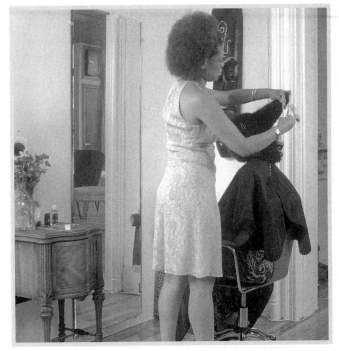

SHAPING NATURALLY
TEXTURED HAIR

hair out. Check your ends or have your stylist check to see if your hair needs to be shaped while you're using these products as a growing-out method.

If you see that one hair shaft is split into two, then you know that you have split ends.

A great cut should have movement, fluidity, and hold the shape from visit to visit. A trim is different from a style cut. A trim involves shaping the hair after receiving a great cut, generally taking off anywhere between an eighth of an inch up to one inch.

The cut is the foundation. Every visit you schedule for a shaping will maintain that fabulous cut. If you stay away from your stylist too long, she may have to recommend a style cut for your hair. At this point, the ends are probably damaged and only a style cut can save your hair, which usually means taking off more than two inches.

When you receive a style cut, you are actually receiving a complete

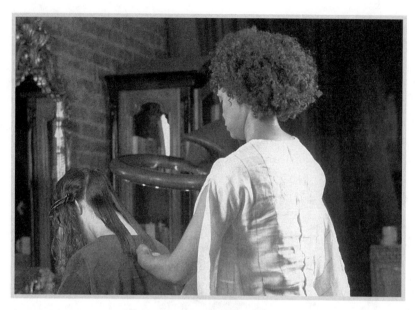

REGULAR TRIMMING
PREVENTS SPLIT ENDS

change in style. And change is always good. If you're ready to receive a great style cut you should keep these helpful reminders handy.

1. The styles that you see on your favorite celebrities aren't always meant for you. So consult with your stylist, taking into consideration your face shape, which is either round, oval, square, or oblong. Your stylist should be able to suggest a cut that complements your face.

2. If you see a great style cut on another woman, compliment her first, then get the telephone number of her stylist. When you look good you feel good, thereby adding to their happiness. So remember to receive the joy and bask in the light.

3. Be mindful of who is cutting your hair. Every stylist isn't necessarily a master precision cutter. A master precision cutter has studied under one of the master cutting houses like Vidal Sassoon, Tony & Guy, Pivot Point, Dudley's, or Bumble and Bumble.

When receiving a cut for very curly and tightly coiled hair, it is very important that your hair is blown out using a blow-dryer and a wide-tooth comb or a pick. This enables the stylist to see the line perfectly and also

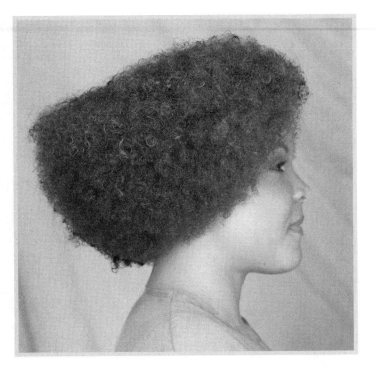

BLOW-DRYING IS THE FIRST STEP
WHEN TRIMMING VERY CURLY HAIR

the split ends that are undetected when hair is wet and curly. A trained eye can see all the lines in any great cut. Once you've received a great cut, any stylist can follow those lines.

Wavy and curly hair can be cut wet, but it is important to cut the hair on the S-curl pattern, using the bounce-back technique to ensure that not more than the amount intended is cut. The hair is stretched out and held straight. Once the amount of hair to be cut is determined, the hair is held loosely and then slowly returned back to its natural wave pattern. The hair should be cut at the end of the S pattern.

Relaxed hair can also be cut dry or wet. However, in my experience, whether the hair is relaxed or in its natural state, when it is cut dry you will receive the best results from a precision cut. Many well-known Madison Avenue salons use this method of blow-drying straight hair and then cutting the hair dry, sometimes even flat ironing first, to achieve a precision cut.

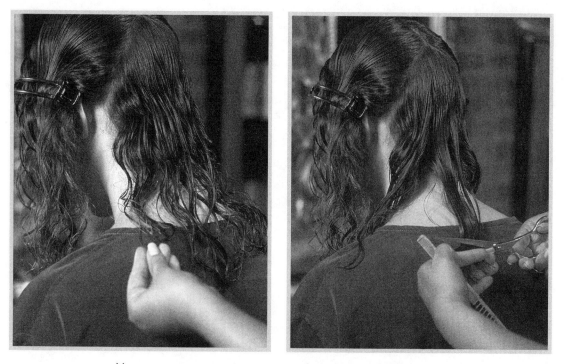

YOUR STYLIST SHOULD LOOK FOR THE S PATTERN BEFORE CUTTING

The most popular method of cutting the hair today is texturized cutting. This technique is used to shape the hair, give it dimension, soften it, and/or create wispy ends. Texturized cutting can be used to remove bulk from wavy hair as well.

Razor cutting, also called slicing and chopping, is another popular method. Slicing and chopping with a razor is also a popular method for blending weaves and curly extensions. Your stylist should approach cutting locs as she would any other style. The only difference is that the strands of hair are thicker and three dimensional. Your stylist should use separate shears for cutting locs because the thickness of the locs tends to dull the shears quickly. She should never be afraid to cut your locs. The technique is the same, the hair just has a different dimensional texture. I've created all types of shapes for my loc clients, from bobs to short layer locs to long layers with flips.

Unfortunately, sometimes you will see hairstyles that are shaved and chopped off in the back and lines that are intrusive. All cuts, shapes, and styles should be blended unless intentionally created otherwise. This is what we call a universal cut. You shouldn't be able to see horizontally chopped lines. Your best bet is to leave the cutting, trimming, and shaping to the professionals.

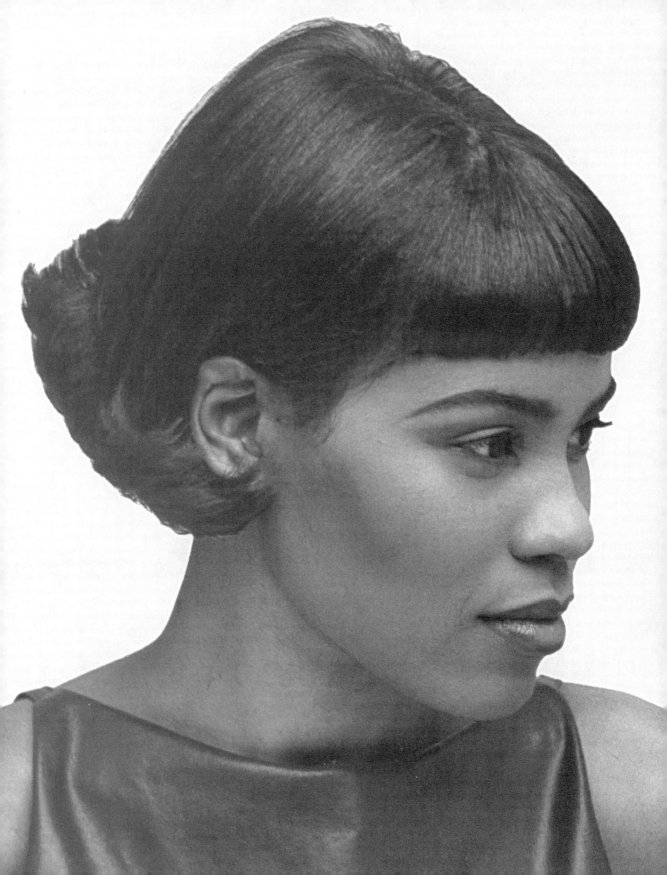

SEVEN

Chemically Speaking

Changing God-Given Texture for Manageability and Versatility

*Textured hair is freedom—a woman having the ability
to wear her own natural texture any way she'd like, be it
relaxed or with a natural wave.*

—Felipe, precision cutter, NYC

I am constantly asked the question "Do chemicals damage your hair?" And I always answer with "What is damage?" Chemicals only alter the structure of the hair. Damage is caused by failing to take proper care of the hair. The chemical process commonly known as relaxing will alter or change your natural texture, breaking down the natural structure of the hair. This process inherently strips the hair of protein, the building block of hair structure. In order to keep your relaxed hair healthy, you must revitalize the hair by replacing what has been taken away.

The relaxer systems today are far more superior than in the past. I *strongly* recommend going to a professional to receive a relaxer, texturizer, or softener (see the Salon Directory). However, for those who feel they must bring out the hair stylist trapped inside themselves, consider having a friend or relative apply the chemicals. This way you're more likely to avoid overprocessing and damage to the hair shaft. Please make sure the instructions are followed carefully and always use the

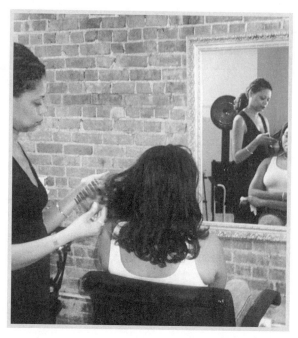

products contained in the system or package. For regular washings and conditionings after your chemical process, feel free to experiment with the products that work best for your hair texture. Again, I recommend botanical products derived from plant and flower essences. Try to stay away from products that contain mineral oil, beeswax, lanolin, or petrolatum (petroleum jelly). Popular styling products that are referred to as waxes are simply product brand names and are very effective in sculpturing and molding textured hairstyles.

There are various types of relaxers and softening products to choose from: sodium hydroxide–based (lye), calcium hydroxide–based ("no-lye"), and thioglycolate-based are just a few. There is also a new Japanese reconditioning relaxer on the market that straightens the hair for up to one year before reapplication is necessary. Touch-ups are applied every three months. However, it's not recommended for highly textured hair; rather, it's for wavy or very loose curly hair. It is comparable to thioglycolates and uses a patented thermal straightener (flat iron) for activation. This method is similar to the Wave Nouveau but instead of restructuring the curl pattern the hair is flat-ironed straight and then neutralized.

No-lye relaxers are actually rather harsh and can be very drying to the hair because they contain calcium as their main ingredient. Although they are usually recommended for their slow processing and gentle treatment, over a period of time their use can result in brittle, dull, and lifeless hair. No-lye relaxers are usually recommended for sensitive scalp applications and color-treated hair.

I've used almost every brand and do recommend the professional lines used by certified professional stylists. Relaxer systems that I recommend for use by your professional stylist are

- Mizani Relaxer System
- Avlon Affirm Fiberguard
- Sensitive by Nature
- Gentle Treatment
- Texture and Tones for Color-Treated Hair
- SoftSheen-Carson (Optimum Professional MultiMineral Relaxer)

When the hair is relaxed 80 percent, not only is this healthier for the hair, but it also leaves a slight wave pattern so that you can wear your hair wavy or straight when heat is applied. Generally, if your hair is relaxed 100 percent you are overprocessing, creating lifeless hair. "Basically what it boils down to is that we have been relaxing 100 percent," says precision cutter Felipe. "If we decide to relax away from the scalp, seventy to eighty percent, we would get a nice wave pattern within that structure. With very good conditioners, this would give you the ability to style and the freedom to wear your hair any particular way."

When the hair is relaxed the bonds are broken and the natural proteins are taken out of the hair. That is why the products that I recommend have conditioning systems that build back the protein in the hair while the cuticle layer is still open, supplying the hair with the proper conditioning directly into the hair shaft. Follow up with a deep-penetrating conditioner.

Texturizing is a special relaxing technique that allows the stylist to achieve a softer, more manageable look with your natural curl pattern. Timing, technical application, and the strength of the chemical (usually mild to normal), depending on your natural curl pattern, are the factors that will determine great results.

A texturizer will release your natural curl pattern, adding softness and sheen to your hair. Texturizing a zigzag curl pattern should result in a soft afro blow-out. However, if the chemical is left on too long, your hair will become straight. In the same way a texturizer can turn a curly pattern into wavy curls, a coily pattern can become spiral curls.

Naturally textured hair may have more than one curl pattern throughout the head. That is why the technique is very important. Also,

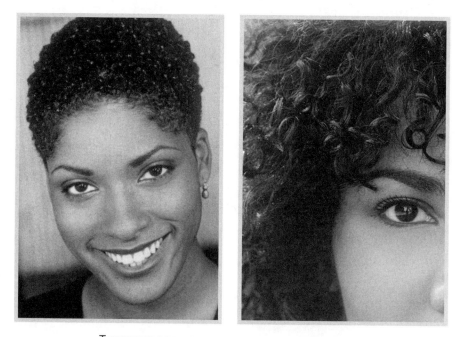

TEXTURIZERS CAN GIVE YOU A LOOSER, SOFTER LOOK

texturizers usually work well with hair that is short or already at a desired length. Generally, it should not be used to grow out the hair unless you have a wavy curl pattern. Why? Because as you continually apply the chemical on the new growth, the rinsing will inevitably cause the product to run over the already texturized hair, straightening the hair over a period of time. The result—no more texture, just straight hair.

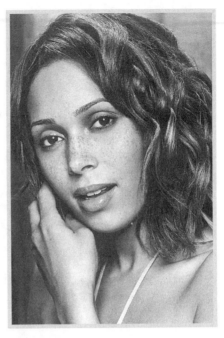

RECORDING ARTIST TAMIA

Softeners (thioglycolate-based) generally work best on hair that is wavy or has very loose curls. When applying any chemical products to hair that has been colored, make sure that they are products specifically developed for color-treated hair, usually marked "for fine and color-treated hair."

Conditioning is the key to healthy chemically treated hair and the steam moisturizing cream bath can be your salvation. (See Chapter 3, Life in a Bottle, for instructions.)

Growing Out a Relaxer

The texture of your hair plays a large part in the method or choice used to grow out the relaxer. Wavy hair is soft and very elastic. Therefore, the wave pattern of relaxed wavy hair will not easily break off. Very curly or tightly coiled curl pattern drastically differs from the now relaxed hair, thus making it more susceptible to breakage when growing out a

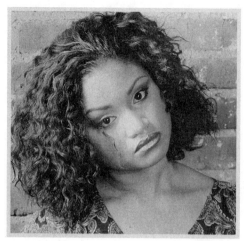

WHILE GROWING OUT A RELAXER, CONSIDER USING A NATURAL SET (SEE CHAPTER 8)

relaxer. Breakage usually occurs after four to five months of unrelaxed time.

Conditioning is always key in growing out any chemical process. Also important are maintaining stressless hairstyles that stay away from added heat applications, and avoiding pulling and tugging especially on the hairline or any area that's held by a hair band or an elastic band.

Thermal Straightening

An alternative to relaxing natural hair to create a straight effect is thermal straightening. Both thermal combs and electric combs are commonly used to straighten the hair at home. I caution those who use thermal combs at home not to abuse this method while trying to keep the edges or, for that matter, the whole head straight. If you choose to straighten your own hair, I suggest that you use a thermal comb with a temperature gauge on a low setting.

The old-fashioned hard press is the method hairdressers used to use to straighten the hair. A hot comb and some pressing oil usually did the trick. While this method left your hair very straight, it also broke down the cuticle layer, leaving the hair thin, lifeless, and damaged over a long period of repeated pressing. It's almost as if you straightened your hair with a chemical. Overapplying heat to the hair by combining blow-drying, pressing at a high temperature, and then curling will result in damage over a period of time.

THERMAL STRAIGHTENING METHOD

1. Blow-dry the hair with a paddle brush or the Denman brush.

2. Apply Carol's Daughter Hair Honey Mimosa Pomade, Aveda Anti-Humectant Pomade, or Aveda Control Paste.

3. Section the hair, then use an electric flat iron to stretch the hair and straighten it flat. Flat irons come in various sizes from thin and small to large and wide. You can purchase a flat iron at any beauty supply store.

4. Barrel curl, flat twist, or plait for a few days, then release and style.

Chemically Altering Your Child's Hair

First let me state that I prefer natural styles over any chemical processes, especially for children. Nonetheless, I recognize that there are parents who must have assistance and insist on using chemicals. I recommend texturizing your child's hair only when the child is able to care for the hair him- or herself or at least understand that daily maintenance is very important after coming from the salon. Generally, I don't recommend relaxing/texturizing until the age of 14 or 15. Keep in mind that your child should only receive a texturizer or mild relaxer—as opposed to a full-strength relaxer—to make the hair more manageable at home. Regular visits to the salon are highly recommended. Consult with your stylist for her professional opinion and get her advice on maintaining your child's hair at home between visits.

I cringe to think about it, but I know there are still those of you who insist on processing your child's hair at home, and you know who you are. Please, please, please always use a kiddy perm and follow the instructions to the letter. I recommend using a mild product such as Gentle Treatment mild strength.

I must reemphasize that a stylist is the best person to care for your child's hair. Although it can be very costly, repairing both your child's hair and her self-esteem after overprocessing is even more expensive.

PART TWO
ACHIEVE IT!

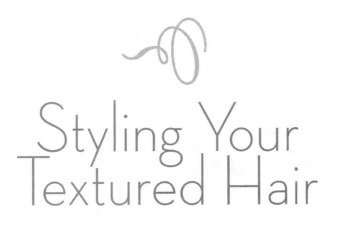

Styling Your Textured Hair

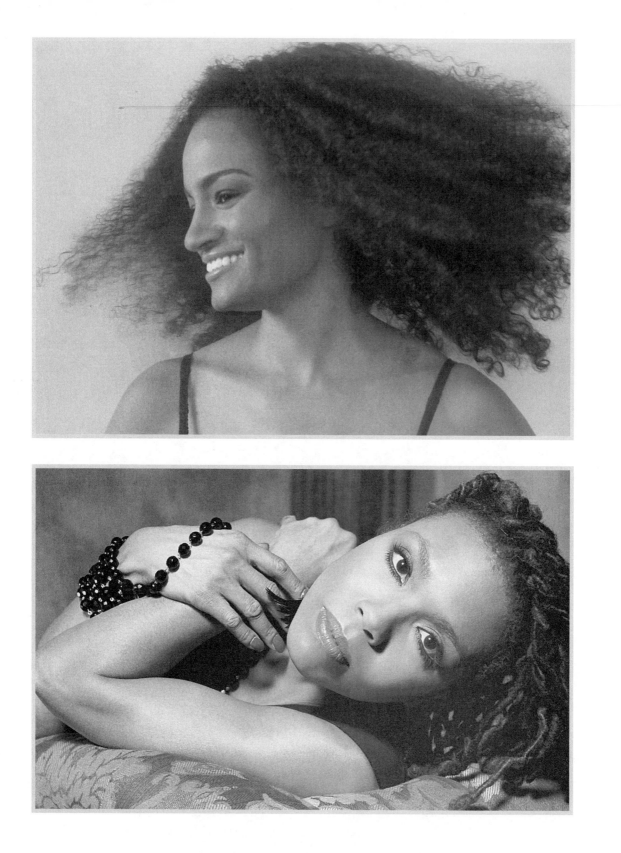

Get Inspired!

Now that you can truly appreciate the beauty of your textured hair, make your hair happy and healthy, purchase the products to maintain your tresses and the tools for proper hair care, team up with the right stylist and salon, make the necessary changes via cutting and shaping, and decide whether to change or not to change your God-given texture with chemicals, we can move on to the fun stuff—styling your textured hair!

For a long time naturally textured hair was viewed as political or bohemian, but rarely ever stylish, versatile, glamorous, or fun. Now everyone, including you, knows better. Natural free hair, twists, coils, locs, and braids are on the red carpet of movie premieres, the Emmy, Grammy, and Tony awards ceremonies, music videos, television commercials, movie screens, and even in the workplace. Your styling options with textured hair are virtually endless. You can set your hair in exotic knots and undo them to wear a funky 'fro. You can rod your two-strand twists for a cute curly look or extend them for a sultry, longer length. Wear your locs and braids straight down during the day when you're feeling more conservative, but pin them up at night and let a couple of strands hang loose for a more glamorous look.

In the pages that follow, I'll show you how to style your textured hair

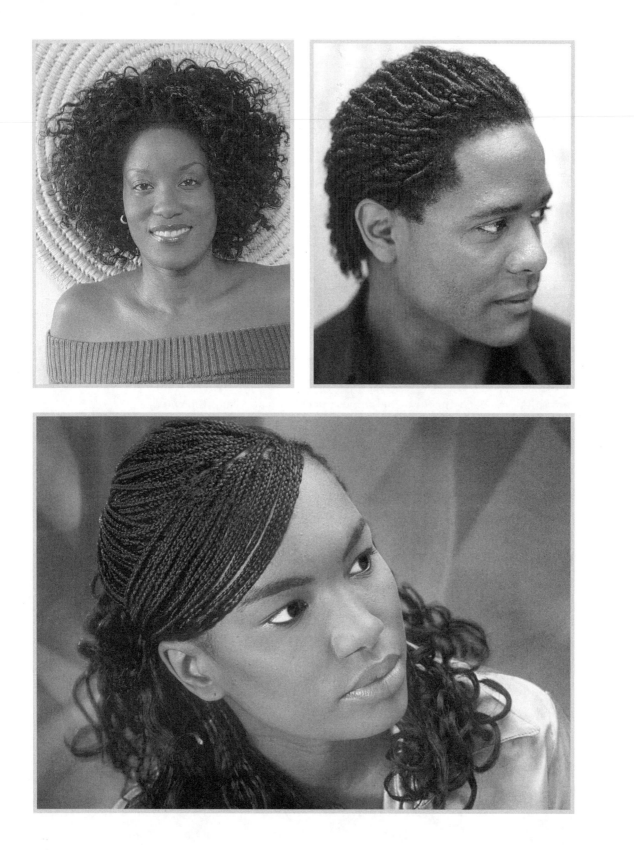

in a clear step-by-step fashion. Also included are timeless, original hairstyles I have created over the years that I call "retro styles." Since this is an era of rediscovery, I refer to the fresh new looks of the retros as "revival styles." I'll even share my personal memoirs with you on what it was like doing a celebrity's hair and then show you how to achieve that exact same style on yourself. Let my styling techniques serve as inspiration for you to create your own masterpieces. Through trial and experimentation you'll soon discover which styles flatter your features and what products work best with your texture.

By the way, who says you have to wear your textured hair in the color you were born with? Who says you can wear only one color with textured hair? Read Chapter 14, The Aura of Color and Illumination, and see how I refute both of those questions. I will reemphasize here as I mentioned in Chapter 5, In Harmony: Picking the Right Stylist and Salon, that coloring is best left in the hands of the professionals, as are some textured styles. While all the styles featured in Part 2 certainly can be done at home, there are certain elements of the styles themselves that require professional input, such as braiding and cornrowing. You may refer to other books that I recommend in the References section for more detailed instructions on these techniques, though I strongly suggest utilizing a hair professional for assistance.

Ready to do it up? Grab your products and tools. We're going to have a ball styling your beautifully textured hair.

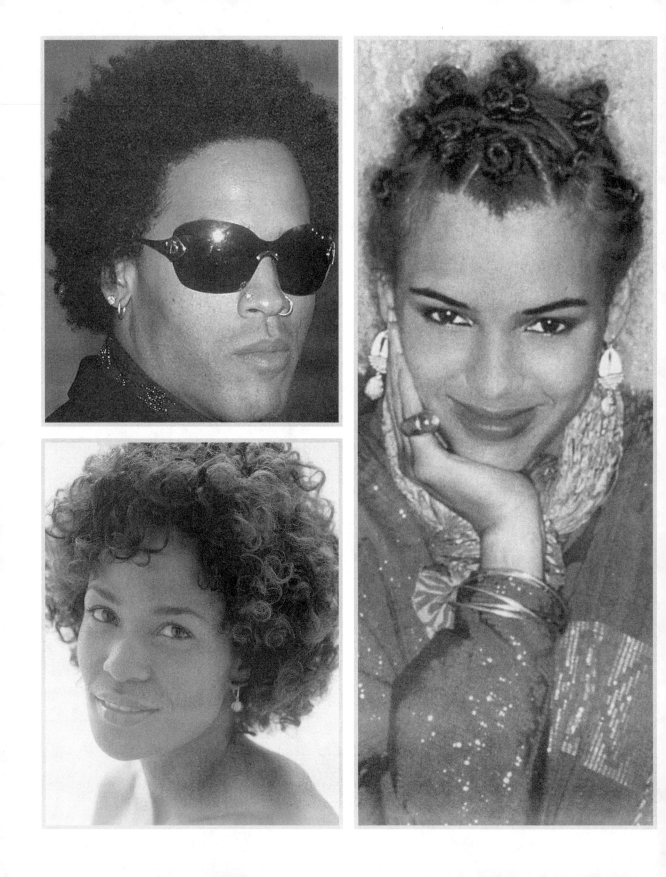

EIGHT

Natural Sets and Styles

Natural free styles allow you to wear your hair loose and free for a week or two without having to shampoo, condition, and apply products on a daily basis. Whether your texture is wavy, curly, or tightly coiled, setting your natural tresses in any of the following sets will allow you to create a free loose hairstyle.

I'll bet you've already attempted to create one of these styles, but somehow it just didn't come out right. Once humidity or any moisture got to your tresses, it reverted right back to its natural texture—shrinking back or frizzing out. Well, ladies, I'm going to let you in on a little secret. The key to getting it right is simply using the right products that work with your hair texture. You'll need to experiment with different products and figure out which ones work best with your hair. However, the products that I mention throughout the book work extremely well on my clients.

Cornrow sets, Nubian knots, plaits, twists, flat twist sets, and spiral rod sets are all popular techniques used to create natural free styles. Cornrows and plaits will create a zigzag curl pattern, while two-strand twists and flat twists will create an S-shape curl pattern. Spiral rods on

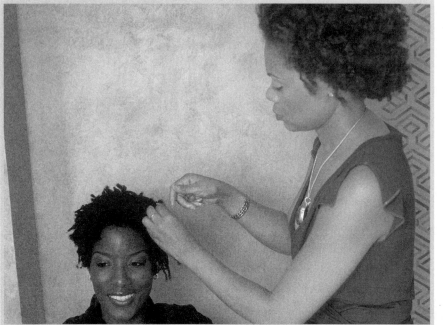

DIANE
STYLING COILS

FLAT TWISTS
CREATE AN
S-SHAPED CURL
PATTERN

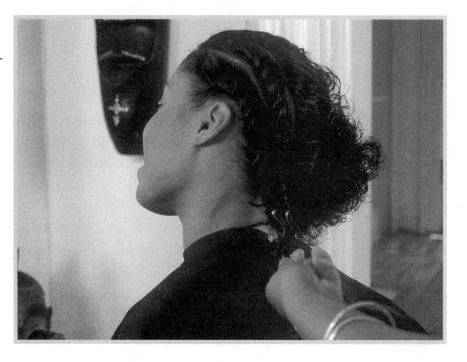

natural hair and long strips of aluminum foil will create more of a coily curl pattern on locs.

Once you have set your hair, get ready to go under a dryer for the long haul or let your hair dry overnight. Whichever drying method you choose, it is absolutely crucial that the hair dry completely before releasing the set.

Once the hair is thoroughly dry, undo the set. Either finger comb or use a style comb to lift the hair for fullness without disturbing the newly created curl pattern. If you skip any of the aforementioned steps, your new curl pattern will be loose and lifeless, have frizzy ends, and last only a day or two.

The beauty of natural sets is in their versatility. The sets themselves can be worn as styles—plaits, cornrows, two-strand twists, and Nubian knots are gorgeous styles in their own right. The released sets become their own free styles. To get optimum wear, consider wearing the set as your hairstyle for a few days, thereby locking in your new curl pattern even deeper. Then undo the set and wear the free style for a week or two.

Revival and Retro Styles

Emi, a hairstylist at Artista Salon and Spa in New York City, wears the revival style of the Ubo knots both as a set and as a loose free style. Nigerian women of both the Ibo and Edo tribes inspired the Ubo knots. Emi is originally from Japan and has been wearing her hair in different textures for the past five years. She's even permed her hair with tight rods to wear a short afro. Currently she sports a curly texture done by twisting and perm waving. Textured hair is a huge phenomenon in Japan. The youths there are using all types of techniques and methods to achieve textured hair—locs, braids, afros, and the like. They even flat-iron nylon strips into their hair to get instant locs. In the retro

REVIVAL

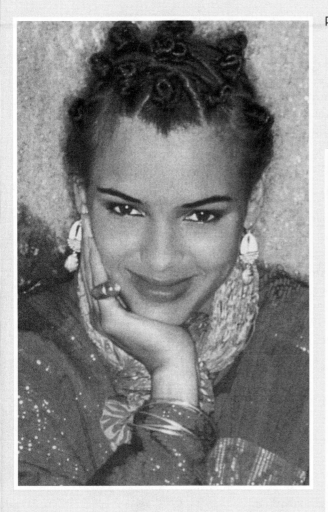

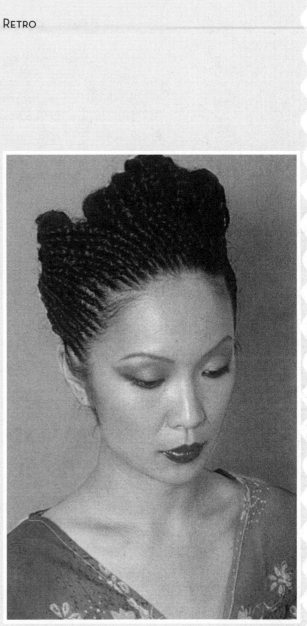

REVIVAL

photo, Tanya wears Nubian knots in a fashion layout for *Essence* magazine with photographer Marc Baptiste. Nubian knots are wrapped tighter than Ubo knots.

Ubo Knots

TOOLS: Hairpins, parting comb, blow-dryer, and diffuser.
PRODUCTS: Aveda Sap Moss shampoo and conditioner, Aveda Phomollient Styling Foam, and Aveda Emollient Finishing Gloss.

1. Shampoo your hair with Aveda Sap Moss shampoo and conditioner.

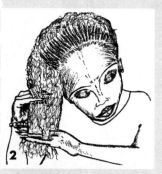

2. Have the perimeter of your hair cornrowed around the circumference of the head three to four inches toward the crown of the head. Apply gel or styling mousse such as Aveda Phomollient to the rest of the hair. Leave hair loose and free for a natural free style look and dry with blow-dryer and diffuser.

3. Parting large sections in circular patterns, take full sections of hair about five inches in diameter creating six or seven sections. Split each section in two. Then twist around the two strands creating an individual Ubo knot.

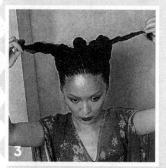

4. Mold the large S-shape twists and form small twists at the ends binding the hair. Tuck the ends under. Secure with a pin if necessary.

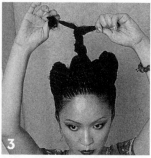

5. Once you've worn your Ubo knots long enough, you can always release them into a free-flowing afro by untwisting knots, fluffing, and finger combing.

6. To wear the Ubo knots as a free style, place under dryer or air dry overnight completely. After drying, untwist and apply a gloss such as Aveda Emollient.

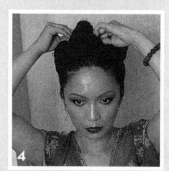

Photographer Jon Peden took the photo of Beverly (see previous page) for *Essence*. Beverly has naturally tight curls, but I wanted to define her curls a little more. Using a medium-sized electric curling iron, I took small sections of curls and wrapped her hair around the iron in a spiral direction, creating softer curls with more definition, minus the frizzies. Even though Beverly's free textured afro is the retro look, her looser defined afro curl is still popular today and will continue to be so.

Nakisha's hair has a much looser curl; however, in the revival style, she achieved the same natural free look by curling with an electric curling iron, separating, and finger combing.

REVIVAL

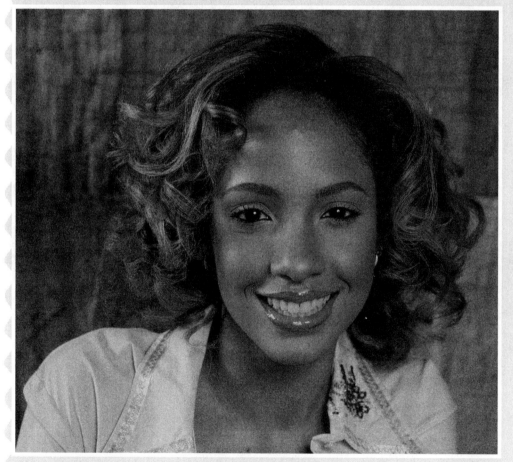

TEXTURED TRESSES

Natural Free Style

TOOLS: Small-barreled electric curling iron and fantail comb.
PRODUCTS: Phyto Rum shampoo, Phytomoelle conditioner,
Phyto Mousse, and Phytologie Défrisant Serum.

1. Shampoo and condition the hair with Phyto Rum shampoo and Phytomoelle conditioner.

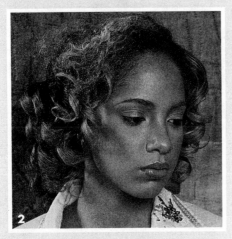

2. Towel dry and apply Phyto Mousse. Allow hair to air dry completely. Now you have your afro, which you can wear for a day or two, reapplying mousse or gel after rinsing daily.

3. To create a softer, more defined look, starting on the right side, separate with a comb or your hands, then pull smaller sections of your textured hair. With a small-barreled electric curling iron, wrap hair around the barrel in a spiral direction.

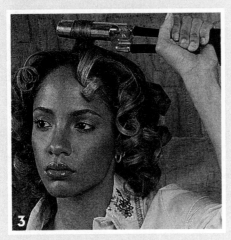

4. Continue throughout your entire head.

5. Now separate each individual curl into two new curls.

6. Continue throughout your entire head.

7. Apply Phytologie Défrisant Serum for gloss.

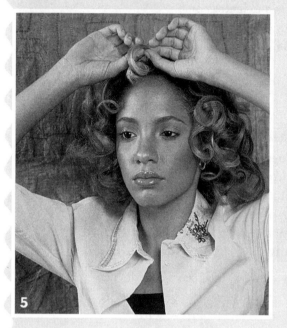
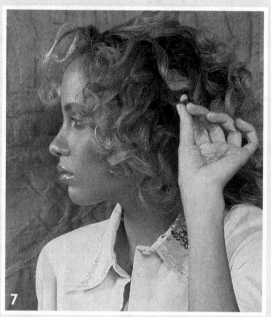

NATURAL FREE SETS

CORNROWS:	Three-strand braiding on the base of the scalp used to create a Z-shape pattern.
KNOTS:	Two-strand twists wrapped into a knot.
PLAITS:	Large-sized braids on natural hair (no hair extensions are added).
FLAT TWISTS:	Two-strand twists created flat to the scalp of the head in rows or panels.
SPIRAL RODS:	Sections of hair wrapped around small or large perm rods.
TWISTS (LARGE):	Large sections of hair twisted into two strands around each other as a set, then released for full S-wave pattern.

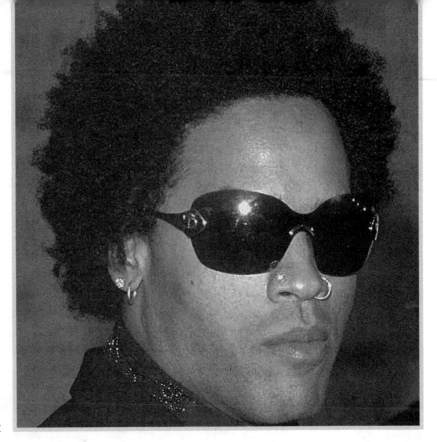

ROCK STAR
LENNY KRAVITZ

Celebrity Memoir
LENNY KRAVITZ

In 1998, Lenny Kravitz called me to do his little girl Zoë's hair in twists. Actually, celebrity agent Bethann Hardison recommended me to Lenny. I'd been grooming her locs as well as those of her son Kadeem of *A Different World* fame since 1994. I met Bethann on a photo shoot for *Essence*.

I went to Lenny's place in Manhattan to twist Zoë's hair. While there, we discussed Lenny's cutting off his locs. Of course I didn't want him to do it. He agreed to come to Dyaspora, my salon at the time, for a steam treatment of herbal essential oils and grooming instead, something he hadn't ever done before. About one year later, after many visits to the salon, he came back with his hair completely short. Of course, I wasn't offended, just a little disappointed that he'd cut off his beautiful locs. However, he was so sweet he felt compelled to explain. He continued to come back for steam conditioning treatment, shaping, and/or cornrows.

One evening Lenny called me to do his hair for the cover of his *Greatest Hits* CD.

He arrived in a limo with his assistant and off to the studio we went. He said he wanted something new and different. We discussed all the possibilities. He decided that he wanted his hair shampooed, conditioned, and after applying moisturizer he would shake his head really hard and get his naturally spiral curls to do their own thing. While on the set I primed, groomed the hair on Lenny's head, and shaved the hair off his chest. Ladies, don't you just love it! I must say he's always a gentleman and very protective of the ladies who work with him. In fact, he always said to me, "Send it [your request] out to the Universe and you'll get what you want."

HOW TO ACHIEVE IT!

TOOLS: Fantail comb, pick, hair dryer or blow-dryer with a diffuser.
PRODUCTS: Kiehl's shampoo and conditioner, pomade, and Kiehl's Creme with Silk Groom.

1. Shampoo and condition with Kiehl's shampoo and conditioner.

2. Apply pomade to the entire head. Use a dime- to a quarter-sized amount depending on the thickness of your hair.

3. Using an angle comb, start at the nape of the neck and make horizontal and vertical parts for each coil.

4. Next, start above the ear on right side of the head, making parts diagonally and continuing to the temple.

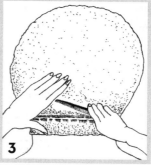

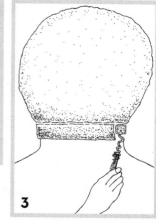

5. Continue on the left side exactly the same way. The rows will eventually cross.

6. At the crown of the head part horizontally. Clip and then coil each section until you reach the front hairline.

7. Sit under a hair dryer for 25 minutes or blow with a diffuser until completely dry.

8. Separate the coils by stretching the ends and splitting the coils up the middle with the fantail comb or your pinkie finger to create two coils.

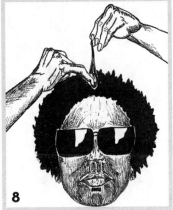

9. Using a pick, place at the base of the hair, right off the scalp, and slightly lift hair for more volume.

10. Apply gloss or oil, or moisturizer such as Kiehl's Creme with Silk Groom.

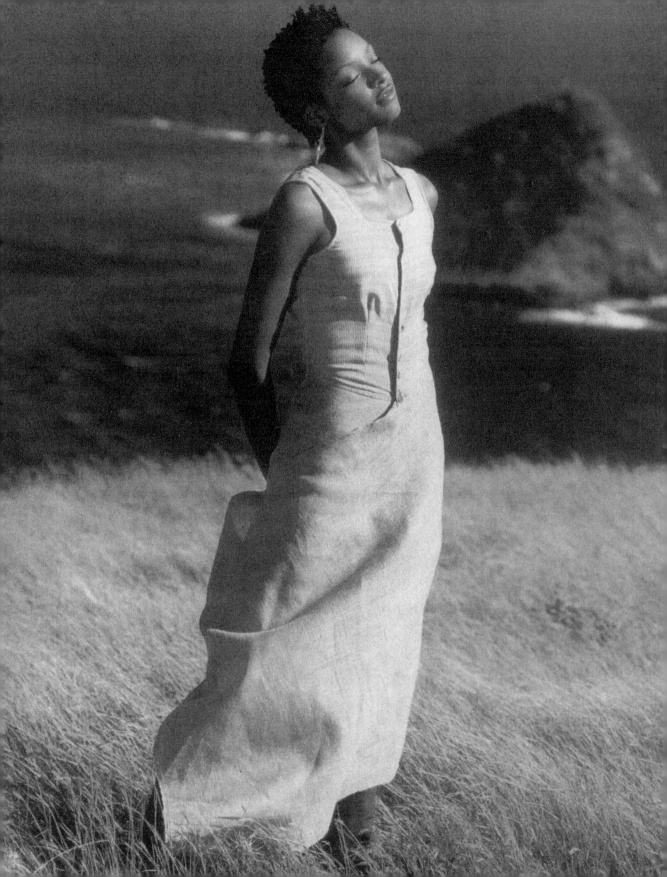

Twists and Turns

Remember when your mother didn't have time to braid your entire head, so she'd whip in a few fluffy twists instead? Sometimes she'd make two big, bouncy, ponytailed ones, other times a bunch of springy, spongy twists wrapped in colorful rubber bands. These are the predecessors to the popular twisted styles you see today on the heads of women of all ages with all types of textured hair—kinky afro twists, curly twists, short twists, long twists, natural twists, and extended twists.

Senegalese twists were the original double-stranded twists created by braiders in Senegal. Extending the hair with Lin fiber or human or synthetic hair creates long-lasting twisted styles.

There are various sizes you can play around with when creating your twists—small, medium, and large. Both small- and medium-sized double-stranded twists can be worn as a twisted style and last up to three weeks, or released the day of the set for a fuller look that can last up to 10 days. Two inches of your own natural hair is enough to twist a full head of hair. Twists can also be used effectively as a method to lock both wavy and curly hair.

Larger twists are generally used as a natural hair set and then released immediately. Twists can also be rodded for a curly effect or roller set for a fuller loose curl. Both naturally straight and relaxed hair can be

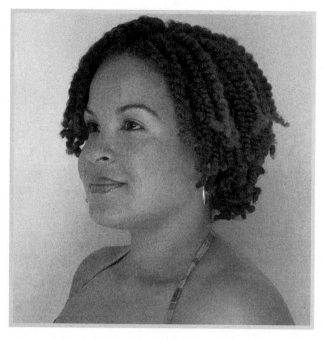

LARGER TWISTS CREATE
FULLER, LOOSE CURLS

twisted with the ends rodded for more hold. Twisted straight hair will last for about seven to ten days.

Leaving your twists in too long, say past four weeks, may result in the beginning stages of locs. The hair will lock naturally if left alone without combing. Keep in mind that proper maintenance assures a long-lasting style. So tie your hair at night with a silk or satin scarf or even a bonnet. Make sure you wear a shower cap when bathing and apply a natural oil or gloss to the hair daily or as needed for moisture and sheen.

Revival and Retro Styles

Malonda Richard wears a beautiful display of Afro Twists in the revival photo. The former BET video host had been wearing her hair in a larger-than-life version of the Twist Out style for more than five years.

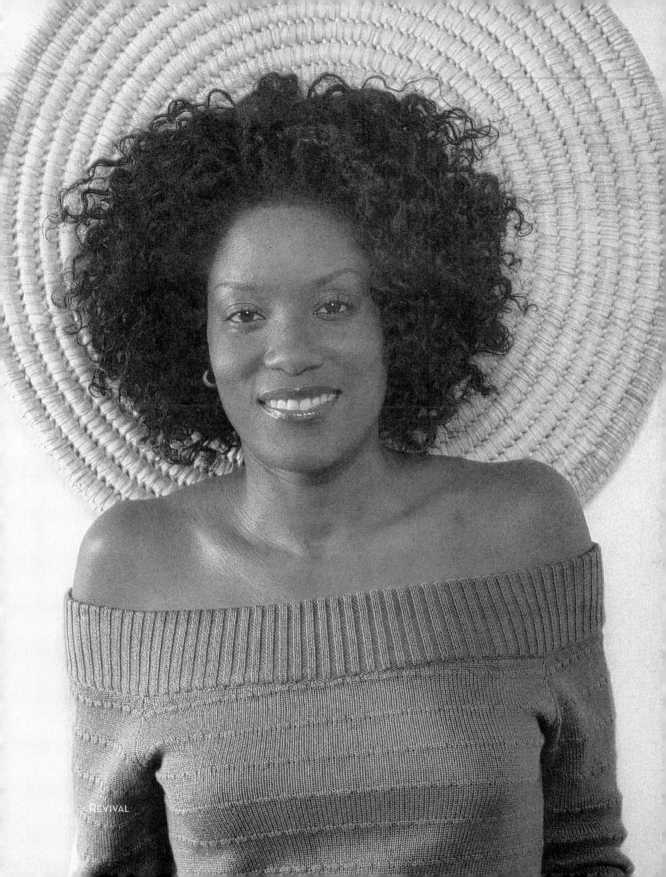

Revival

Her hair was literally so huge that people would stop her on the street. Malonda even told me that the BET executives once called her into their offices because she'd trimmed her signature Twist Out 'fro a bit too much.

On a recent visit with me at Artista Salon in New York City, I discovered that Malonda's hair was hungry for some much-needed attention and conditioning. She'd been experimenting with colors and texturizers. She knew a cut was long overdue but had been avoiding it. Though I'd explicitly explained to her how much I'd have to cut off, she was a bit shocked after her trimming. Her hair had never been this short.

Malonda came to the photo shoot with a weave done by Hadiiya Barbel for Studio 1 in Brooklyn, New York. I asked Hadiiya to twist Malonda's weave into individual two-strand sections and then release them once the hair was completely dry to achieve a more natural look. Now Malonda can sport this Afro Twist look while she nourishes her hair from the inside out to keep it healthy as it grows.

The Twist Out was my first natural hairstyle that appeared in *Essence* magazine and put me on the map. This style was so popular that I was booked three months in advance. It was nearly impossible to get an appointment with me. I traveled the world on this hairstyle. The "Essence" Twist Out was created with very small, double-strand twists, dried for 20 minutes, then untwisted after the hair was completely dried. This ensured that the wave pattern would have a beautiful S-shape curl without frizz. I lifted the hair in an upward direction with a tortoiseshell comb to achieve extra fullness.

TEXTURED TRESSES

The Twist Out

TOOLS: Wooden wide-tooth comb, fantail comb, butterfly clips, hair clips, spray bottle, blow-dryer with diffuser.
PRODUCTS: Aveda Brilliant Humectant Pomade or Aveda Control Paste, Carol's Daughter Mint Shampoo and Lavender Rinse, Mimosa Hair Honey, and Tui Oil.

1. Shampoo and condition with Carol's Daughter Mint Shampoo and Lavender Rinse.

2. Emulsify a quarter-sized amount of Carol's Daughter Mimosa Hair Honey in the palm of your hands, smoothing the Mimosa over the entire head.

3. Part the hair into four sections: top crown, both sides of the head from back of ear to the front of the hairline, and the complete back section. This will enable you to move freely and quickly when parting your individual sections. Section and hold with butterfly clips.

4. Starting at the back section, create a horizontal part from right to left. Use a clip to separate the larger portion of hair from the parted section.

5. Apply a dab of pomade or paste to each section as you proceed.

6. Now section off one inch for each section as you vertically part the hair.

7. Take the one-inch section and split the hair into two more sections. Holding each section in both hands, cross one section of hair over the other section to create a double-strand twist. Then place a silver or plastic clip on the twist for control.

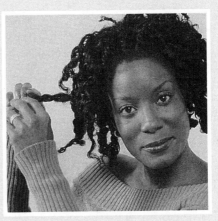

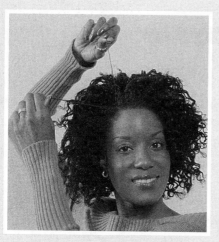

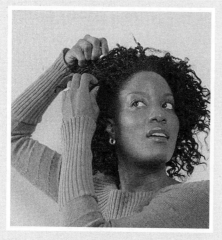

8. Continue this pattern until you reach the crown of the head. The crown section is where you determine the direction of your hair, whether you want your hair to lay completely back or fall to the side of your face.

9. Blow-dry with a diffuser or sit under a hooded dryer for 20 minutes. After the hair is completely dried, untwist each twist one by one.

10. Take each individual twist and separate into two twists.

11. Apply a dime-sized amount of gloss, like Aveda Light Elements Smoothing Fluids, to the palms of your hands and sweep the hands over the head in a back and forth motion.

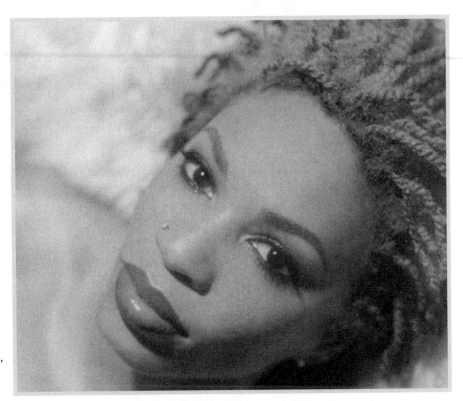

Celebrity Memoir
CINDY BLACKMAN

Lenny Kravitz referred Cindy to me. Cindy Blackman is one of the baddest drummers on the planet. Just ask Lenny. She's his drummer. In fact, Lenny brought Cindy to my salon specifically to create a new style for his *Lenny Kravitz 5* CD tour. He wanted her to cut all her hair off, but Cindy wasn't going for that. So he asked me to create some sort of afro-looking style that looked like the 'fro she'd been wearing on stage. I thought I would have to weave her hair, but Cindy wasn't going for that, either. So I created a braided style with spiral Afro Curl extensions. They were both happy with the results.

Cindy had been coming to me since Lenny first introduced us. After wearing the braided style, Cindy wanted to wear her hair natural. So we started playing around with color. I colored Cindy's hair a golden blonde, which made her inner spirit glow even more. She wore her colored twists for almost three years, as seen on the *Someday* CD.

Before getting both her color and twists redone, Cindy would release them and wear the Twist Out. The fullness and color looked just great. Every time she walked in or out of the salon, folks would stare. She was beaming.

Cindy is an accomplished jazz percussionist in her own right. When she isn't performing with Lenny, she's busy recording, traveling with her own band, and teaching music to a group of children. At one point I hadn't seen Cindy for quite a few months while she was touring. By the time I saw her again, her ends were begging for a trim. I sensed some hesitation but didn't understand why at first. Apparently, Cindy had a bad experience with another hairstylist.

Unfortunately, I actually had to cut more of Cindy's hair than she desired. She wanted her hair to remain a certain length since she had been growing it out for so long and it had come so far. Needless to say, she was very upset, but didn't let me know until the very end of our session. And boy, did she let me have it.

"Diane, I want explicit instruction on how to care for my hair when I'm not able to come and see you," she said. "If you tell me what to do, I'll do it, because I want my hair to be healthy. When I teach my students to drum, I do this, and that's what I expect from you." So I did. I told Cindy exactly what she had to do to care for her growing hair. She needed to condition, condition, and condition. Plus she needed to get her hair trimmed regularly and use some of the products that I use in the salon on her hair at home. I recommended Carol's Daughter Tui Oil for an herbal hot oil treatment under a heating cap or in a sauna once a month. I suggested shampooing with Aveda Shampure and conditioner every two weeks, along with using Aveda Curessence conditioner to stop any breakage.

Communication is always the key to understanding and relating to all clients, whether they are artists, entertainers, or hardworking everyday individuals. I was so sure that was the end of Cindy and me. But guess what? She came back. Cindy eventually decided to grow out her color and wear her hair free and natural, moving toward that textured afro look—the very same look that Lenny got excited about when he first brought her to the salon. After growing out the color, she experimented with two-dimensional color, meaning more than one color: the natural color of her new growth with blonde color enhancement on the ends. This look is very popular in Europe.

While attending the World Hair Show in London, I noticed that everyone was wearing this "under color," which is two shades of color, a darker tone underneath from the ear to the nape of the neck and a lighter color in the crown area. No one was really wearing it in the United States, so Cindy decided she would work this style for a while and give her hair a rest. Today Cindy's hair is happy, healthy, and long.

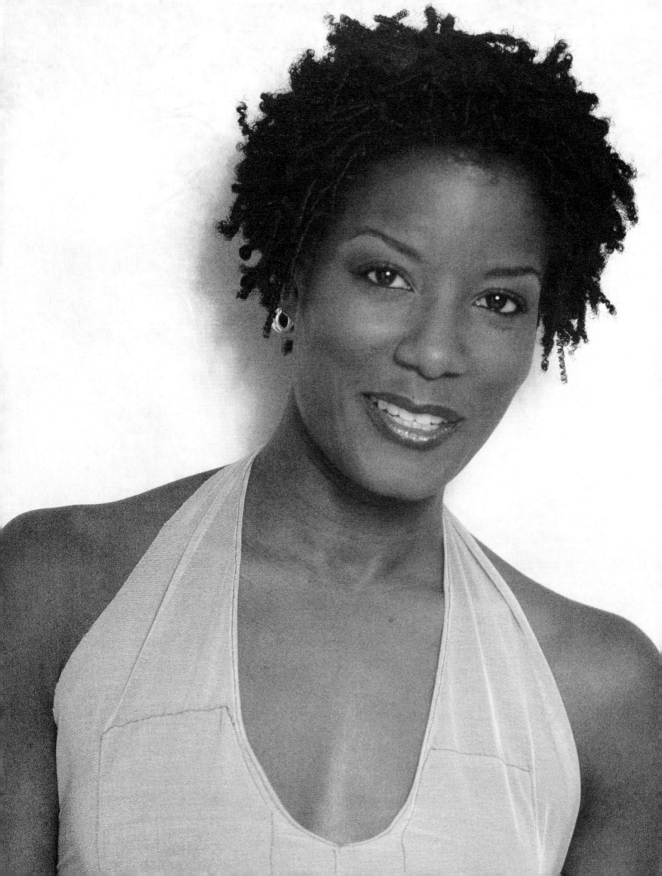

TEN

Coils and Curls

Coils are the alpha and the omega, the beginning and the end. They can be worn as a fabulous style, or as the genesis of locs. You can start coils with just a few inches of textured hair. They offer a stylish, yet conservative means of wearing very curly and tightly coiled textured hair, particularly after growing out a chemical or a short cut.

On the other hand coils can represent a committed, maybe even permanent way of life and style. As the first stages of locking hair, coils can be traced back to the Egyptian technique of spinning the hair, using the hands as tools. In fact, while visiting the Brooklyn Museum of Art, Ona Osirio Maat, "The Locksmyth," was inspired by Egyptian artifacts. Paying special attention to the placement of the hands in the depictions of ancient Egyptians locking hair, Ona learned to form twists into "spools of thread," using the hair itself to fill up the circumference of each coil.

Remember the Shirley Temple curls on the good ship *Lollipop?* Those were large, loopy coils that Shirley Temple wore, created by roller setting her hair in a spiral set. Today, wrapping curly hair around a fantail comb or spinning individual strands around your index finger can easily achieve those very same curls.

Pictured here are the curly coils achieved by wrapping two to three coils around perm rods, resulting in a tightly coiled effect.

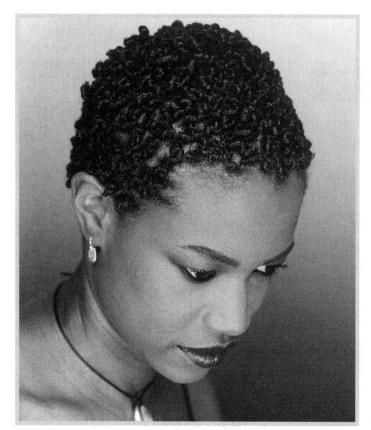

Revival and Retro Styles

Nanya Akuka Goodrich sports the gorgeous Twisty Coils in the revival photo. The actress and singer usually wears her hair natural and free. Her spirit exudes her presence.

Janine Green wears the retro coils while playfully swinging through a bed of daisies. Peter Ogilvie photographed Janine's coils originally for *Essence*. I worked with Janine on various *Essence* projects and she frequented the salon for coils quite often. She is one of the first models to sign with a major color company wearing her hair naturally textured in a variety of colors.

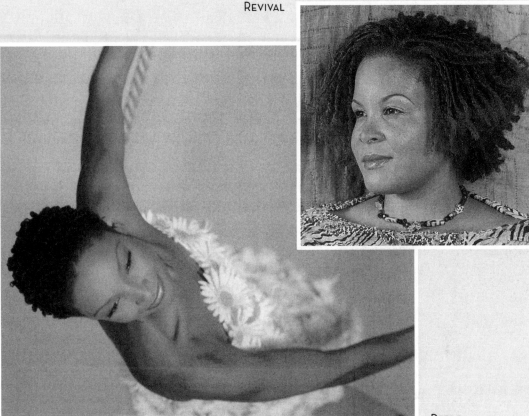

HOW TO ACHIEVE IT!

Twisty Coils

TOOLS: Angle comb, hair clips, hooded dryer or blow-dryer with diffuser.
PRODUCTS: Carol's Daughter shampoo and conditioner, Carol's Daughter Mimosa Hair Honey, Lisa Elixir Oil.

1. Shampoo and condition hair with Carol's Daughter shampoo and conditioner.

2. Apply a quarter-sized amount of Carol's Daughter Mimosa Hair Honey over the entire head. Continue to apply as needed throughout the styling process.

3. Spray hair with a bottle mixed with half water and half lavender oil. Keeping hair moist, continue to apply as needed.

4. Starting at the nape of the neck, part one-inch horizontal rows. Next, make a one-inch vertical part. Rest the narrow edge of the angle comb on the head. Holding the end of the hair, twirl your wrist in a circular motion with the comb flat against the head to create a coil. This is the comb/coil technique.

5. You can also use the hand coiling method. Instead of a comb, use your index finger and thumb as your tools. Pick up and separate individual sections of hair, then twirl them around your fingers to create coils.

6. Clip your coils down with hair clips as you continue, until you reach the crown area. Use this same method on the left and right side of the head. As you approach the forehead, clip and angle coils to the side.

7. Once you've completed your entire head, sit under a hooded dryer for 30 minutes.

8. After your hair has completely dried, your coils will lie flat and have a neat appearance. Apply Lisa Elixir Oil on hair for moisture and sheen.

9. Take each coil one by one.

10. Now separate each individual coil into double coils, creating a fuller and spiral affect. *Voilà!* The Twisty Coils!

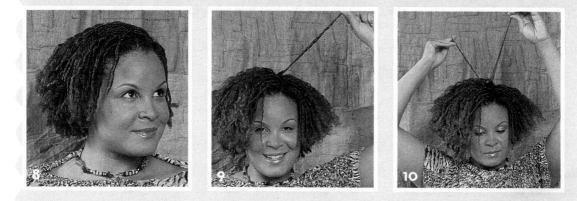

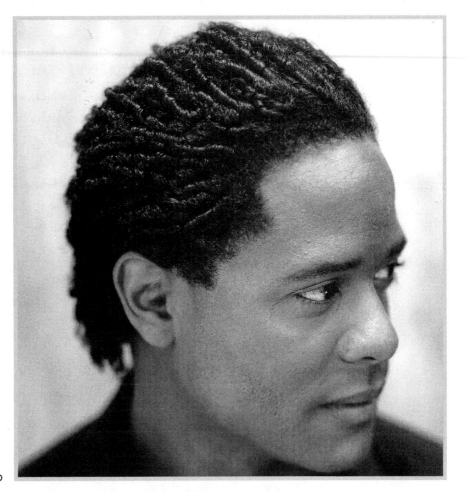

Celebrity Memoir
BLAIR UNDERWOOD

Two nights before Blair Underwood would arrive in New York City for the filming of the movie G, I received a phone call from him. "I'm shooting this movie in the Hamptons and I'm wearing my hair in this twisty thing," he said. "I've been doing it myself and I'd like to wear my hair free and natural when I'm not working. I want your expert advice on what my options are and how else I can achieve this look for the movie."

Of course I was more than honored to do Blair's hair. We met at Sam Wong

Salon in SoHo, where Blair got his first professional natural textured style. My creative direction inspired him to style his hair this way using either a straw set or by washing, conditioning, applying hair products, shaking his head, and wearing his hair freely. He told me recently that he's been wearing his hair like this since the first time he came to me for G. While visiting me at Sam Wong, Blair also received the ancient Chinese secret massage, a deep invigorating finger shampoo massage followed by a luxurious lavender oil head, neck, and shoulder massage courtesy of Yin, a wise assistant at Sam Wong. Would you ever want to get up off that table? Well, neither did Blair.

HOW TO ACHIEVE IT!

Blair is pictured with a straw set coil that he wore in the movie *Full Frontal*, with Julia Roberts, August 2002.

> TOOLS: Spray bottle, parting comb, straws or spongy perm rods, and hooded dryer.
> PRODUCTS: Aveda Shampure shampoo and conditioner, Aveda Brilliant Humectant Pomade, Aveda Styling Curessence, and Aveda Brilliant Shine Spray, Aveda Brilliant Emollient Shine, or Aveda Light Elements Shine.

1. Shampoo and condition hair with Aveda Shampure shampoo and conditioner.

2. Apply a quarter-sized amount of Aveda Humectant Pomade over the entire head. Continue to apply as needed throughout the styling process.

3. Spray head with a bottle filled with a mixture of half water and half Aveda Styling Curessence. Keeping hair moist, continue to apply as needed.

4. Starting at the nape of the neck, part one-inch horizontal rows. Then, make one-inch vertical part. Continue this method on both sides of your head.

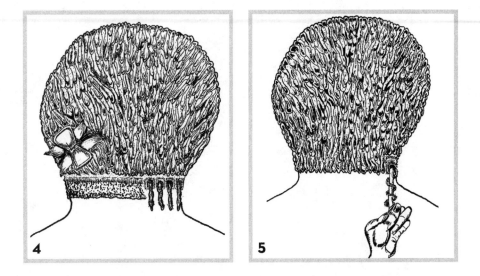

5. Wrap the parted hair section around straws or a long, slim, spongy perm rod in a spiral direction.

6. Sit under hooded dryer for 30 minutes.

7. Carefully remove straws or rod.

8. Spray with Aveda Brilliant Hair Sheen or apply Aveda Light Elements Shine with the palms of your hands in a back-and-forth motion.

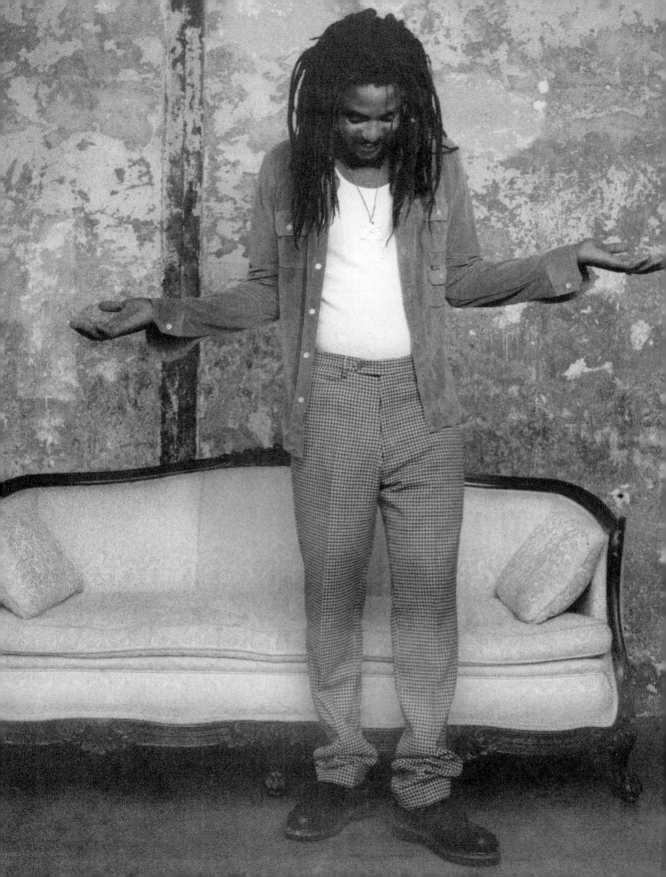

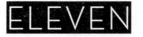

ELEVEN

Locking and Tightening Up

Locking comes naturally to me. When I was just a young girl, my mother would coil my sisters' hair with a large comb. Curious about hair, I tried it out on myself. In the late 80s, I began locking in the salon with the comb/coil method. As I perfected my techniques, I developed many different ways of locking hair, depending on the texture. Although I've been inspired by various stylists' techniques, I was most impressed with Ona the Locksmyth of Locksmyths Hair Groomers in Brooklyn. Her salon specializes solely in starting, grooming, and styling locs. Ona uses an Egyptian-inspired loc technique. This locking process is done without clips to hold the hair in place while grooming and palm rolling the hair.

Young people wear their hair in locs for many reasons. For some it is a spiritual awakening; for others it is a trend. They grow it long, then cut it off and move on to the next style in the blink of an eye. If you're not watching, you may miss the experience.

When it's time to release the energy and start anew, most spiritually inclined people will let go of their locs and go short, perhaps to start again or not. Those of you who love the styling aspect of textured hair

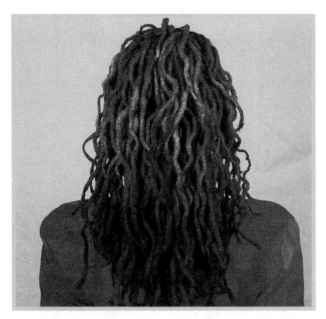

should experience the array of beautiful designs your stylist and even you will be able to create for yourself.

Locs are a creative and beautiful way to wear your natural hair in a carefree and easily maintained style. They originated in both Kenya and Tanzania with the Samburu people, who are related to the Massai Mara tribe. Before becoming warriors, the boys in those regions prepared each other's hair by twisting and applying an ochre red clay mixture to the hair.

Still, it was the legendary reggae singer Bob Marley whose free-spirited locs were most influential in creating a universal appeal for locs. The term "dreadlocks," though frequently used and often associated with Rastafarians, is misleading. As many natural hair care professionals will tell you, there is absolutely nothing dreadful about wearing your hair locked. On the contrary, locs are symbolic of strength, freedom, and ease.

Bethann Management founder and owner Bethann Hardison decided to lock her hair because it freed up her time to concentrate on more important things such as developing her mind and spirit and creating a financial foundation, rather than dealing with daily styling dilemmas. "Now it is just style," says the former model.

Growing your hair from baby locs to full-length locs can be a very spiritual experience. It is a very nurturing and caring process. Locking your hair is also a serious commitment. However, it can also be fun and stylish. You can flip them, roll them, wave them, and cut them in various styles.

Coiling or twisting the hair when it is about two inches long creates baby locs. This is the first step in growing your locs. Exceptional stylists can catch hair as short as one inch long but most will ask you to start with closer to two inches.

Next is the budding stage, when your locs begin to form a bundle of hair within the coil/loc itself. The hair usually starts budding toward the end of your loc, and as your loc grows the bud will spread in an upward and downward direction. Though locs are soft at first, you'll know your hair is locking when the many strands of hair start shaping into a hard cylinder formation.

Locs tend to be dry and brittle because the natural oils from your scalp are not reaching below the midshaft to the ends of your locs. Therefore, it is very important to moisturize your locs with natural oils on a daily basis or as needed.

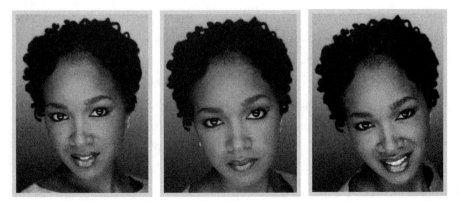

COILY LOCS

Depending on its texture, hair starts locking in one to four months and may take as long as eight months to a year to lock completely. Regardless of whether the hair is straight, wavy, curly, or tightly coiled, all hair will eventually lock.

Free natural locs (think Lenny Kravitz or the reggae singer Yami Bolo on chapter opening page) are grown without retwisting or grooming the new growth. These locs should be washed with a detoxifying peppermint or mint shampoo followed by a lavender rinse and an herbal oil mixture scalp massage. Some clients actually prefer to apply only aloe vera and a steam treatment to moisturize the hair.

When applying the herbal oils to your locs, gently separate the new growth. This process is a very important step. It will prevent your locs from tangling and matting together. Naturally textured hair will hold together and form locs on its own. The natural curl pattern will intertwine between the curls and form knots, resulting in locs. After wearing locs for at least seven years you will find your locs naturally snapping off at the ends. You can either let them go naturally or simply have them shaped and groomed by a professional.

I've started locs using various techniques: the comb/coil, twisting, braiding, hand coiling, as well as loc extensions. All methods use palm rolling for follow-up sessions and maintenance. Here's a breakdown of the various locking techniques.

Comb/coil technique: achieved by placing an angle-cutting comb on the scalp and twirling the hand and wrist in a circular motion to create coils or Shirley Temple curls. Small, medium, and large locs are determined by starting the width of the parts between ¼ to one inch.

Hand coiling technique: similar to comb coiling. However, instead of a comb you use your index finger and thumb as your tools.

Twisting techniques: creates locs by separating a parted section of hair into two sections and intertwining each section around the other, creating a rope effect.

LOC GLOSSARY

FREE NATURAL LOCS:	Locs that are unstructured and naturally groomed (not in a salon).
TEXTURED LOCS:	Created by braiding, cornrowing, knotting, or flat twisting and then releasing for a wavy effect.
LOC SET STYLES:	Created by setting locs with cornrows, plaits, and knots and wearing your locs as is.
STRUCTURED UPDOS:	Elaborate swept-up styles usually secured with pins.
CAREFREE LOOSE UPDOS:	Achieved by gathering loose locks and tying or knotting them freely around each other. May be tied on top of the head or all over.
GENILOCS:	Created by braiding and wrapping the hair with yarn.
YARN LOC EXTENSIONS:	Extensions created by braiding and wrapping the hair with yarn. Originally seen in Africa as elaborate styles created with string wrapping.
SILKY LOCS:	Created by wrapping synthetic hair around an extended braid to create a shiny loc effect.
HUMAN LOC EXTENSIONS:	Created when afro-textured human hair is wrapped around an extended braid for a more natural effect.
SISTER/BROTHER LOCS:	Tiny knots created with a crochetlike hook needle. Works on any texture hair—straight, relaxed, or tightly coiled.

Braiding technique: braids are used to create locs when the hair is very fine or straight. The hair is plaited individually in different sizes, again according to the size you would like your locs, and then secured at the ends with an elastic band or with wax pomade.

Loc extensions: achieved by various methods with either synthetic locs, afro human hair, or by sewing on locs previously cut off. Typically, locs can be prepared beforehand with a palm rolling technique and then sewn right onto the scalp. Braiding the hair and then wrapping with either synthetic or afro hair can also create extensions. Loc extensions require a very long and tedious procedure. Any stylist using this method should be fully compensated for their work. Prices usually start at $1,500.

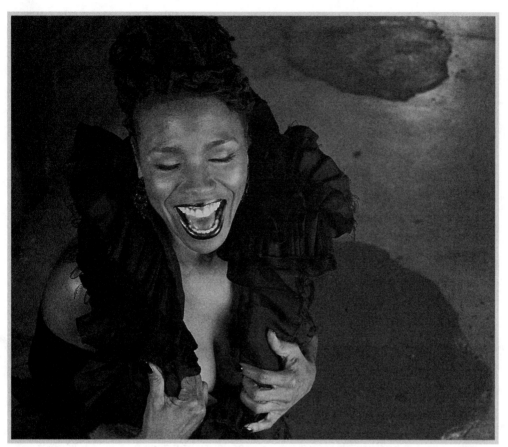

Revival and Retro Styles

The Twist Loc updo worn here by jazz singer Dee Dee Bridgewater is a revival of the retro style featuring the model Michelle taken by renowned photographer Matthew Jordan Smith. I created Dee Dee's hairstyle at the photo shoot for her latest CD, *This Is New*. Dee Dee is both an electric and exciting singer and person. She has worn every style you can imagine, from a short blonde Caesar to locs with purple and blonde attachments.

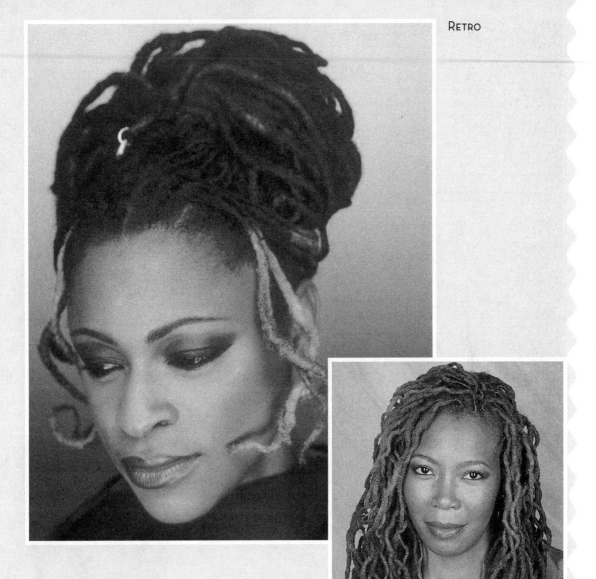

DENISE MARIE
BEGINNING WITH SHOULDER-LENGTH LOCS

This retro look was first featured in *Sophisticate's Black Hair Style and Care Guide*. First, I highlighted Michelle's locs with a multi-dimension color, then roller set her hair and swept her locs to the center of her head, securing them with a band at the crown. Next, her locs were spread out to give them a funnel effect, and secured with hairpins.

Locs

TOOLS: Spray bottle, large clips or butterfly clips, and hair pins.
PRODUCTS: Paul Mitchell's Tea Tree shampoo and conditioner, lavender oil, frankincense oil, jasmine oil, Carol's Daughter Mimosa Hair Honey, and Carol's Daughter Khamit Oil.

Denise Marie will show you how you can create Dee Dee's look at home.

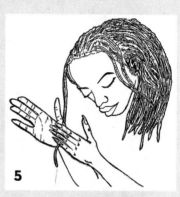

1. Shampoo and condition your hair with Paul Mitchell's Tea Tree shampoo or Carol's Daughter Mint shampoo and conditioner.

2. Spray your head with a bottle filled with equal parts lavender oil, water, frankincense oil, and jasmine oil.

5

3. Next, apply Carol's Daughter Mimosa Hair Honey to the entire head.

4. Starting on the side or the back of the head, separate each loc with large clips or butterfly clips while leaving a few rows free.

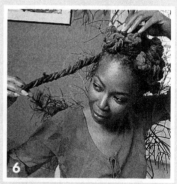

5. Palm roll your hair by taking each loc between your hands and let your one hand move upward and the other down.

6

6. After you have completed the entire section, gather six to eight locs together and twist them. Holding the end of your loc, twist and twirl until you create a knot, then tuck the end underneath, securing the knot. Hold with a pin if necessary.

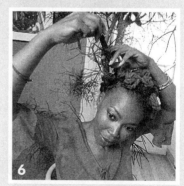

6

7. After the hair is completely dried, release each knot to create a newly formed S pattern in your locs.

8. For the updo, which is very easy to achieve, simply separate a row or panel, diagonally parting across the head to create a sweeping effect.

9. Flat twist against the scalp, holding the end of the locked twist and making circular motions to create a very loose large knot. Secure with a pin. Continue this technique on the entire head.

10. Toward the back of the head you can vertically section your locs, clip away, and continue upward to the crown.

11. Finish with Carol's Daughter Khamit Oil.

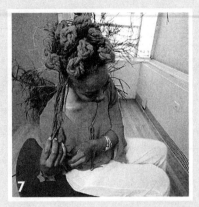

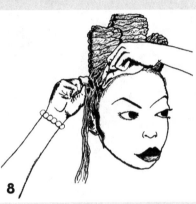

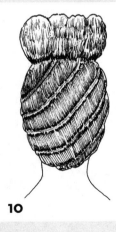

Jazz trumpeter Roy Hargrove

ROY HARGROVE

Grammy Award–winning jazz trumpeter Roy Hargrove first came to me while I was still at Turning Heads Salon. Discovered at his high school in Dallas, Texas, at the age of 17 by Wynton Marsalis, Roy has recorded 12 CDs, with a new funk CD *Hardgroove* featuring R&B wonders D'Angelo and Erykah Badu. At age 19, Roy sported a High Top. I've taken him from light to dark fades, to dark Caesars, to his current shoulder-length locs. In fact, I've restarted Roy's locs at least three times. I cut them at one point simply because he was feeling shorter locs.

My fondest memory of Roy is his visit to me after his return from Germany. He had a lot of "travel energy" in his hair and he wanted his locs washed and retwisted. He started preaching the gospel and said his whole life would change from that day forward. On another visit back from Istanbul, he spoke of chanting and of his daughter, Kamala. He said hair was a symbol of his strength and that he never wanted me to trim or cut it again. Nonetheless, his locs must always be cleaned, groomed, and styled, especially after he comes off the road.

I always cut or groomed his hair for his CD covers right before the shoot. For the *Strings Moment to Moment* CD cover I was able to create something with a little more dimension. Roy always lets me do whatever I want with his hair. I cornrow his locs, twist them, plait them, and for the cover I gave him a crimped loc effect. First I washed and conditioned with herbal steam treatment. Then I groomed and cornrowed them in the salon and the next day went on the set to style his locs. I did Roy's hair and makeup for this CD.

Roy is usually a quiet, humble, and peaceful man, but on stage or in front of the camera, the leader in him appears. This is one artist I love with all my heart.

HOW TO ACHIEVE IT!

TOOLS: Spray bottle, large clips or butterfly clips, and hair pins.
PRODUCTS: Paul Mitchell's Tea Tree shampoo and conditioner, Natural Root Organic Stimulator Tea Tree Oil Pomade, and Lavender/Jojoba Oil.

1. Shampoo locs twice with Paul Mitchell Tea Tree shampoo, then condition with Lavender/Jojoba Oil for 15 minutes with steam from the hot shower. Keep locs loose and free.

2. Emulsify a quarter-sized amount of Natural Root Stimulator Tea Tree Oil Pomade in your hands and massage into the scalp and hair. Apply more if needed.

3. Start from the nape of the neck. Section back area horizontally with butterfly clips.

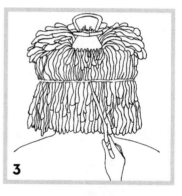

4. Start from the right side to the left side by taking one loc at a time and sliding fingers upward along outer shaft from end to base of the loc. Twist around your thumb and index finger three times.

5. Place the loc between the palms of your hands and roll the loc, one hand up, the other down. This is called palm rolling.

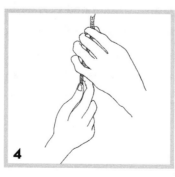

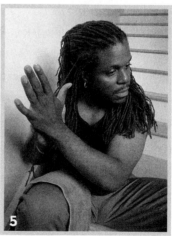

6. Place silver clip at ends of loc to hold groomed loc away from ungroomed locs. Continue panel by panel on each side and crown of head. Bring away from the face, clipping as you palm each loc.

7. After you complete the entire head, section locked head vertically and cornrow each section into six to eight cornrows, binding the ends with elastic bands. Place under dryer for 20 to 30 minutes, then release cornrows for crimped effect. Roy usually leaves his cornrows in for a couple of days or until he's ready to perform, then he'll take them out. Apply lavender oil as needed.

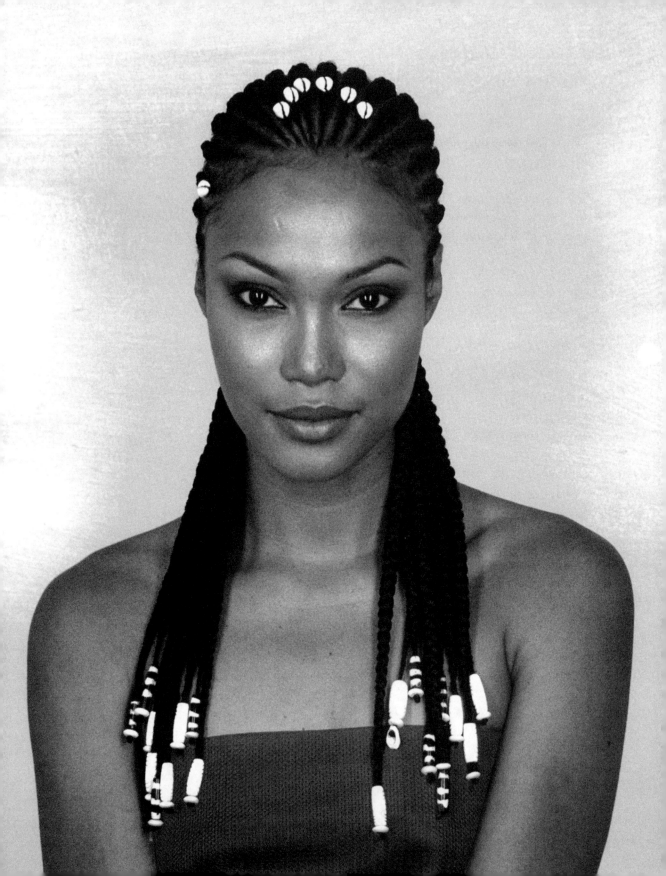

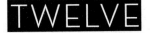

TWELVE

Braids and Weaves

B raids and weaves are two wonderful ways to create new styles. Both give you the opportunity to add length to your natural mane. Even more important, braids and weaves give your own hair a healthy opportunity to rest, grow out a relaxer, and add fullness and body to your tresses. In fact, I've been wearing various braided styles and weaves for the past year while I grow out my own hair for more length.

According to Bethann Hardison, models wore weaves in the fashion industry both to protect their hair and to maintain work. "It gave them versatility," says the owner of the modeling and entertainment firm Bethann Management. "It was birthed out of the fact that it was just easier. Not just easy for the [model], but easier for the hairstylist that had been hired for the job. Models no longer had the problem of the hairstylist not knowing the stylist or understanding our texture. Weaves helped the models fit in. They didn't have to look at their hair take abuse anymore.

"It's interesting to see with weaves, how they became something," says Hardison. "Once [models] started using weaves, the stylist became conditioned. The quality of the hair became better, much better. The girls could afford to really get the best weavers. The stylists who were weaving became better practitioners. The average woman doesn't have

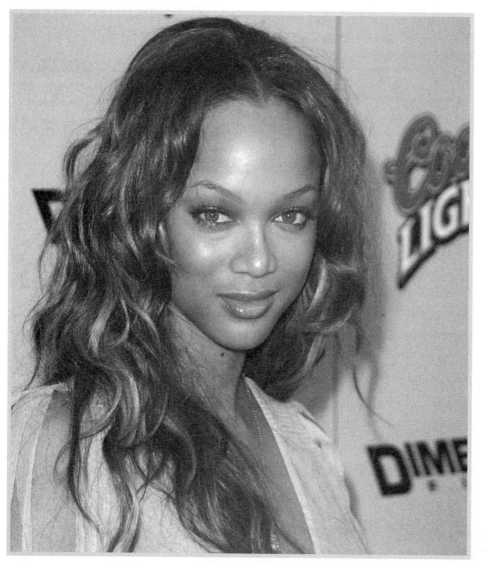

natural full-bodied hair. If she is an actress or a model she has options. But the majority of them wear weaves. She had options, but she chose the weave."

First and foremost, I strongly recommend that you choose your master braider and weaver very carefully. Make sure that they are professional and accommodate you in a clean and aesthetically pleasing environment. Your braider and/or weaver should also be concerned with

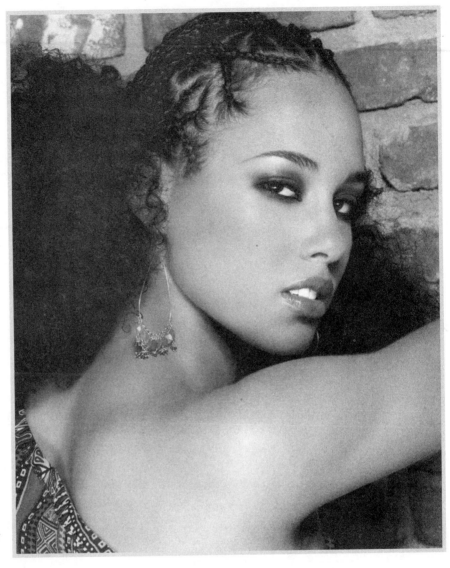

RECORDING ARTIST
ALICIA KEYS

the health of your hair and scalp, not just the style of your braids or
weave. He or she may be a natural hair care specialist/braider or cos-
metologist/weaver.

Braids and weaves come in various sizes, styles, and techniques (see
sidebar, page 136), and can be done with either human or synthetic hair.
I prefer human hair for my clients. It's healthier for the scalp and gives
them a much more natural look.

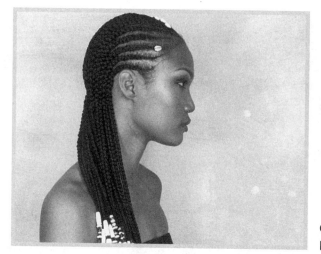

CHEROKEE BRAIDS BY
KHAMIT KINKS

However, synthetic hair does have its benefits, especially for children and young adults. Braids created with synthetic hair can last anywhere from six weeks to two months, depending on the style. However, synthetic hair should not be washed. Instead, mist braids with a mixture of half water, half Aveda Styling Curessence or half Infusion 23, or a mixture of water and lavender oil.

Cleanse the scalp with a dry shampoo such as Bumble and Bumble's Dry Shampoo, or create your own by pouring Carol's Daughter Mint Shampoo on a damp cheese cloth and massaging the shampoo gently on the scalp. Rinse scalp with another piece of damp cheese cloth until entire head is free of shampoo. Massage light oil on your scalp or spray on natural herbal oil that's free of any petrolatum or mineral oil for daily moisturizing. Try Aveda Light Elements Reviving Mist containing lavender and other essential oils.

When washing braids created with human hair make sure you wash your hair in the shower with a mild shampoo diluted with 50 percent water. Place a quarter-size amount of shampoo in the palm of your hands and massage gently, only on the scalp. Let the shampoo run down the entire braid, cleansing the remaining length while preserving your design.

Remember to wear a shower cap while bathing if you are not washing your braids. At night, wear either a satin or silk scarf or even a satin

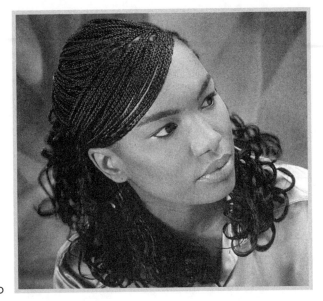

INDIVIDUAL STYLED BRAID

bonnet to protect your braided style. Before going to bed, massage your scalp with light oil such as jojoba or carrot oil for blood circulation and to enhance the natural flow of oil from your scalp to your hair. This is especially important since your hair will not be brushed or combed on a daily basis.

Some stylists recommend that women of color not wash their hair more than once a month, particularly when it comes to natural styles and braids. This may be true in their experience. However, I believe that the condition of your scalp, diet, and lifestyle will determine how often you wash your hair, particularly if you work out, perspire a lot, retain moisture in the scalp, or have any of the scalp challenges I discussed in Chapter 2, Healthy Hair Is Happy Hair.

Generally speaking, I recommend shampooing and herbal steam conditioning your braids every two to three weeks with touch-ups for your braids as recommend by your braider in the salon. Your braids will always look freshly done until your next complete visit.

Contrary to popular belief, if your head is aching and feels very tight during the braiding process or afterward, this is a clear indication that your braider is pulling too tightly on your scalp, which may ultimately

BRAIDS

INDIVIDUAL EXTENSIONS:	Formerly known as box braids, separate loose braids that move freely. May be braided to ends or left loose. Can be created using either human or synthetic hair.
MICRO BRAIDS:	Very small individual braids. Usually done with human hair.
CASAMAS:	Large individual braids.
CORNROWS:	Braids that are attached to scalp in rows.
CHEROKEE:	A style of long cornrows.

result in traction alopecia, or balding in certain areas of the scalp. Bumps and little white pimples are the result of too much tension being applied on the hair and scalp. If this occurs, braids should be removed immediately. The neck muscles and spine may also require massages and sometimes chiropractic adjustments if severe injury results. I cannot stress enough the importance of choosing a master braider and/or natural hair specialist to avoid such negative results.

Revival and Retro Styles

Matthew Jordan Smith took the retro photo of Jenny. I created the large youthful ponytails for Dyaspora Salon publicity photos. Jenny's hair is thick and straight, so her braids or large plaits were secured by elastic bands and left loose at the ends for a fanned-out effect.

In the revival photo of Linda, I created what looks like an intricate style, but really is quite simple to achieve. Linda is a student at Penn State University and a model. This was the first time she had had her hair braided. She was a little nervous at first. However, halfway through the braiding process she let me know that she really liked it.

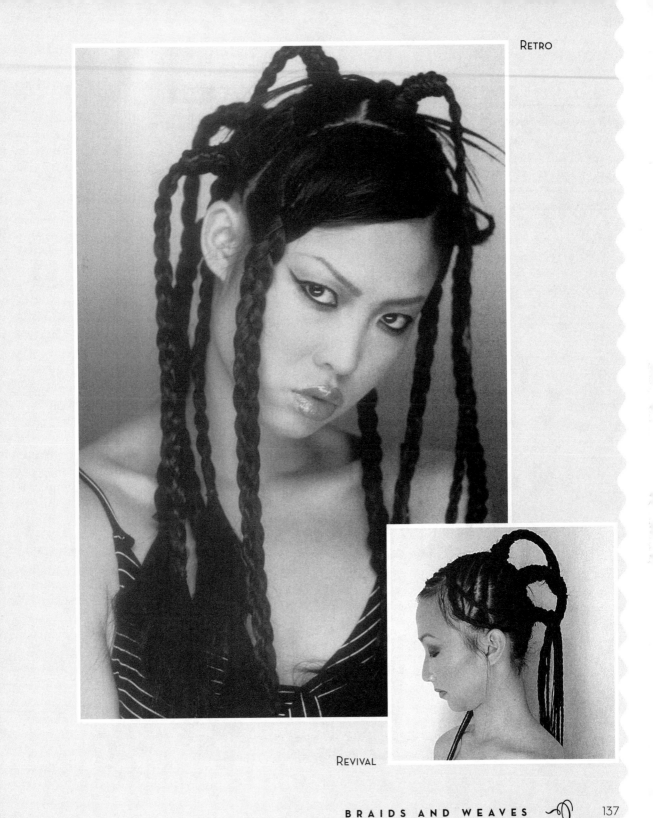

REVIVAL

BRAIDS AND WEAVES 137

Youthful Ponytails

TOOLS: Large bobby pins.
PRODUCTS: Phyto Cleanser and Phyto Light Balm,
or Neutrogena T-Gel Shampoo and Conditioner.

1. Shampoo your hair with a detoxifying/cleansing shampoo such as Phyto Cleanser and condition with a light conditioner such as Phyto Light Balm. Remember to choose the proper shampoo and conditioner for your hair type—oily, normal, dry, or damaged/overprocessed.

2. Have a master braider cornrow your hair from the mid-crown to the front hairline. Then have her put individual braids in the back area with synthetic Kanekalon hair. Finish ends of braids by hand if your hair loosens.

3. Now, take a few braids from the top section and twist them around two or three times. Place a large bobby pin between the braids and stick it into the crown of the head.

4. Repeat on second ponytail.

5. You have created a Two-Loop Ponytail. Let the remainder of the braid fall freely.

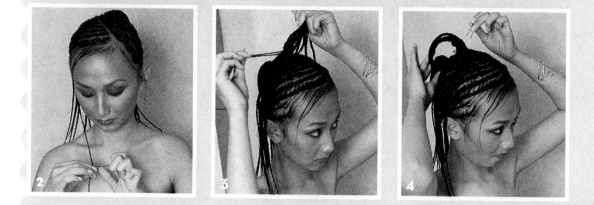

Weaves

Weaving is simply attaching additional synthetic or human hair to achieve fullness, length, and an overall healthier look. Weaves may range from $350 to $2,500.

During the summer of 2002, all the weavers were telling me about the latest craze, the Quick Weave. It was so fascinating. Women were enjoying a quick and safe way of achieving different styles, custom designed by their stylist directly onto their heads.

ADD LENGTH AND FULLNESS
TO YOUR NATURAL HAIR

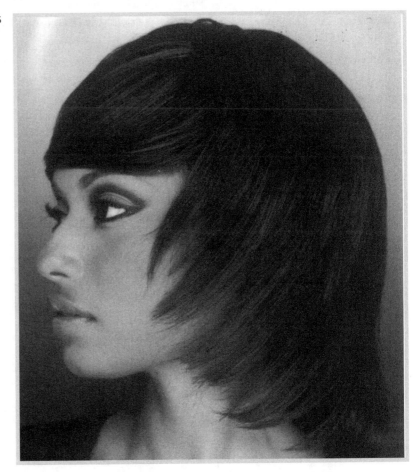

WEAVE GLOSSARY

STANDARD TRACK WEAVING:	The hair is cornrowed to create tracks. Wefts of hair are then sewn into tracks. This method works well on tightly coiled hair.
TREE BRAIDING:	Individual hair strands are picked up and braided right into the cornrow.
STRAND BY STRAND:	Micro weave tied directly to the scalp for invisible detection.
BONDING:	The quickest weave method. Silicone glue is placed on wefts of hair, then the wefts are placed as close to the scalp as possible. Should look flat and natural looking. Works well with straight and relaxed hair.
FUSION:	Silicone glue is applied onto a weft of human hair and then the weft is applied to the base of the scalp with a heated small flat iron.
INFUSION:	The same as above; however, this method is done with strands of hair as opposed to wefts.
FUSION ON THE WEFT:	Silicone glue is applied to the weft and the weft is applied directly to the scalp. The hair is in close proximity to the scalp.
EUROPEAN WEAVE:	Clip or glue-based individual strands of hair applied to the hair on the head with a heating device like a slim flat iron.
MICROEXTENSION:	The weave is done with strands of hair individually tied in knots for an invisible effect. This is a very long and expensive process.
INTERLOCK INVISIBLE:	The hair on the weft is sewn directly to the base of the scalp with a flat roll technique.
INTERLOCKING WITH LATCH HOOK:	Individual human hair is hooked into a base cornrow with a latch hook needle.
KNOT WEAVE:	Created when individual pieces of hair are knotted together and sewn to the base.

Quick Weaves are bonded weaves created by professional stylists who completely wrap your head as a set with a foam wrap lotion. After drying, wrap strips are placed around the entire head to protect the hair while the weave is being bonded. Your stylist then places a nylon weave cap or net cap with spaces for scalp ventilation over your wrapped hair. Next, your stylist actually bonds the hair directly onto the cap on your head. It's quick, easy, and very creative. Absolutely any style can be achieved—straight, wavy, curly, long, or short. How ingenious!

Snap-on weave pieces come in very handy when you want to add length and fullness to your hair. Just take the snap-on comb and have it sewn onto your weft of hair by your stylist. Then have your stylist shape and style the new hair.

It is important to maintain the condition of your natural hair, regardless of texture, when wearing weaves. Usually, weaves should last only six to eight weeks. Full weaves and tracks should be touched up biweekly, depending on the method.

Weave Pointers

Conditioning treatments should be done before, during, and after your weave. Keep your scalp healthy by massaging and oiling it with herbal and botanical oils, unless the weave was done by bonding or fusion. Take care not to remove your own hair when taking out your weave. Shape your natural hair at regular intervals to keep your ends healthy.

For More Information: Book Recommendations
Braiding by Diane Bailey, Milady Publishing, 1997.
Wigs, Weaves, and Extensions by Toni Love, Delmar Publishing, 2001.

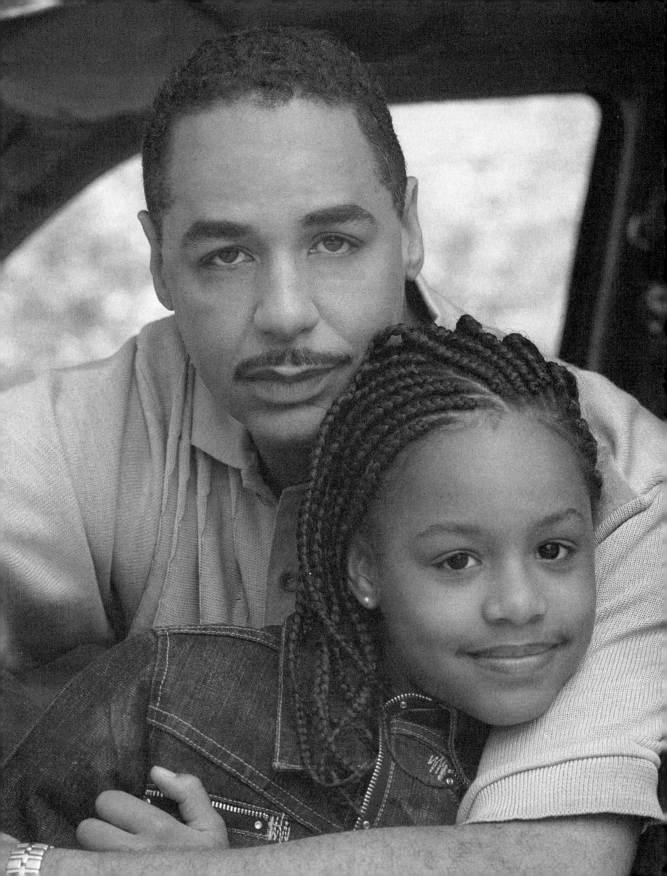

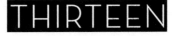

THIRTEEN

Textured Hair for the Family

Textured hair is freedom. Textured hair is versatility. Look around you. Women are not the only ones sporting textured hairstyles. On the contrary, textured styles are for the entire family. Free natural styles, coils, locs, twists, and braids can be worn and are being worn by young and old alike. Textured styles know no gender, financial, or age barriers.

I decided to include a family section in my book to show both the versatility and the freedom of textured hair, to show you that textured hair will not limit you in your profession or your place in life. I have a cross section of clients wearing naturally textured hairstyles—from the wonderful everyday hardworking mother, to the television news personality, musician, art director, and high-powered real estate broker. Textured hair is not only worn by the "creative types" or the "free-spirited" kind. Textured hair is also being embraced by professionals and executives in very prestigious positions throughout corporate America. Their love for their naturally textured hair and styles is being shared with their children, spouses, co-workers, and business partners.

Flip through the following pages and allow me to introduce you to my extended families wearing their textured hair proudly.

Motherly Love

Elizabeth's naturally wavy hair was curled with an electric barrel curling iron, making large soft waves. Using a boar bristle brush, I swept the hair to the sides and secured the hair with a soft elastic band. The soft waves then cascade along her shoulders.

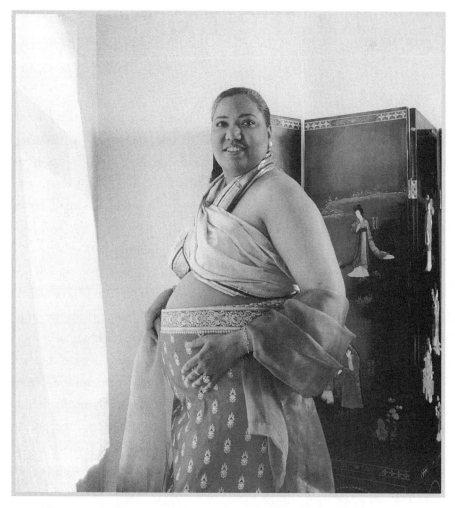

ELIZABETH L. MARTIN, PROPRIETOR AND REAL ESTATE BROKER, AND BABY

Daddy's Girl

Ed Gordon is always well groomed. Just some brushing and lining of the nape was required. I applied Aveda Brilliant Emollient for sheen.

His daughter, Taylor, has a layer of extension cornrows on the crown section. I parted her hair diagonally and added individual braid extensions to the back.

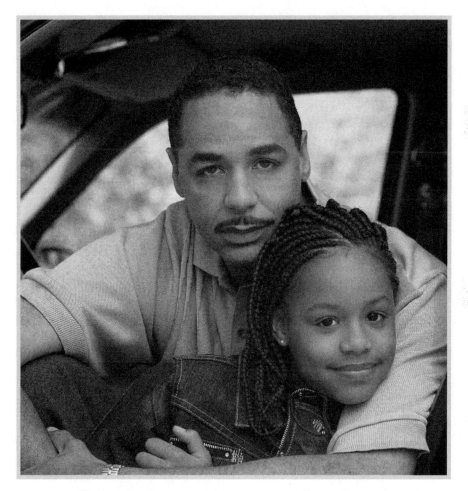

ED GORDON, BROADCAST JOURNALIST, AND TAYLOR GORDON

Mama's Boy

Deidre's naturally curly hair was shaped and then softened with a medium-sized electric curling iron, creating large waves and fullness.

Nine-month-old Evan's young hair is soft and very curly. I applied humectant pomade with my hands and created individual coils by wrapping them around my fingers.

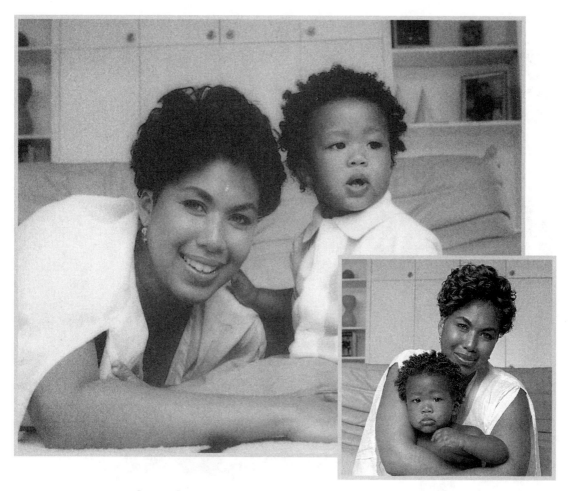

DEIDRE POE, REAL ESTATE BROKER, CORCORAN GROUP, AND EVAN POE SANDERS

Like Mother, Like Daughter

Genny's locs were palm rolled and groomed with Aveda Humectant Pomade right on the set. I touched up her color a few days before with a light brownish amber. On the set she wore her locs in a loose free style.

Kara, on the other hand, was a much lengthier task. Her beautiful tight curly hair was a handful under our time constraints. I styled her entire head in individual twists and then gathered the twists into a top-crown ponytail.

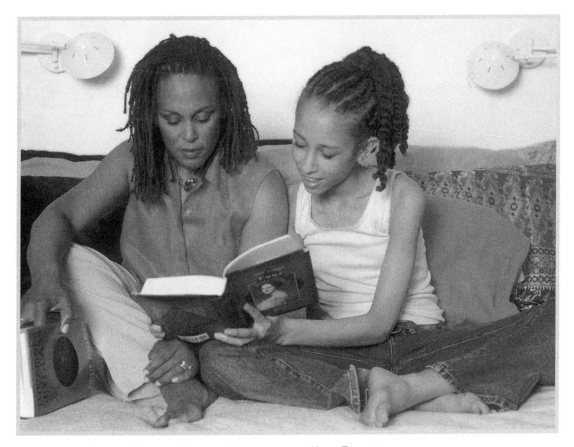

GENIEVA KELLAM, CREATIVE DIRECTOR, AND KARA FOWLER

Forsaking All Others

Leon normally wears his natural hair texturized and slicked back into a ponytail. For this photo shoot he agreed to wear his hair loose and free. I texturized his hair and then braided it into eight large cornrows as a set to wear a few days before the shoot. On the set, I released his cornrows and styled, applying Aveda Brilliant Emollient for shine.

His beautiful wife, Chelsea, has soft, fine, naturally curly hair. Humidity is always a big challenge for her texture. Using Aveda's Humectant Pomade, I coiled individual sections by wrapping strands of hair around my fingers and twirling them into little coils for a neat and professional look.

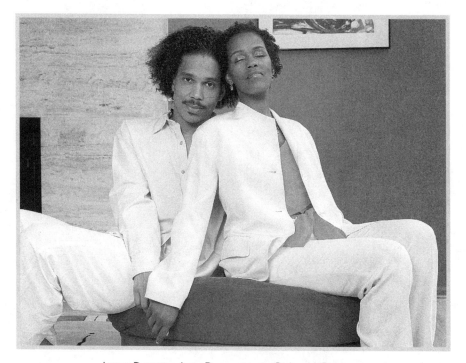

LEON DORSEY, JAZZ BASSIST, AND CHELSEA DORSEY,
PRESIDENT (COO) OF ACCESS.1 COMMUNICATIONS CORP. (WWRL, NYC)

FOURTEEN

The Aura of Color and Illumination

Color will bring out the light that already exists inside of me. My aura will shine with a positive attitude.

—Diane Da Costa

Your hair color should reflect your aura, which comes from your personal light that shines from within. Heavy? Not at all. Think about it. By definition, color is basically the quality of an object with respect to light reflected by it. Color is what makes that brown-skinned sister sporting rich burgundy-tinged hair look so deliciously warm in the fall. It is the reason why that fair-skinned sister looks delectable with hints of orange and blonde tresses in the summertime. A col-

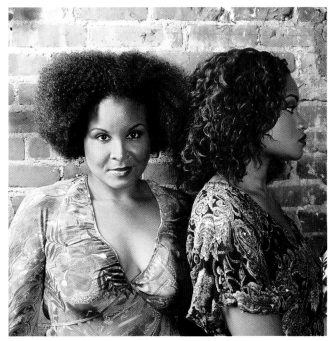

COLOR ENHANCES YOUR NATURAL BEAUTY

149

orist can only enhance your color so that your own natural beauty will shine even more so.

In the fashion industry, there are basically just two seasons: fall and spring. In the hair and beauty industry, we honor all four seasons by creating new colors for each one. It is not unheard of to change your hues and tones for every spring, summer, winter, and fall. Change is inevitable and exciting, both for those who desire just a subtle change from season to season, and for those who want more dramatic change.

In order to see color we have to start with three basic elements—a light source (natural sunlight or artificial light), a healthy set of eyes, and a healthy head of hair. Often women of color with naturally textured hair have very porous hair. Therefore, it is important to condition textured hair before, during, and after the color process with an herbal/botanical steam treatment in addition to a color refreshing conditioner and a deep penetrating conditioner, which will preserve the intensity of color between visits to your salon. If you want to obtain shiny hair color with a high-gloss finish, you must start with a healthy cuticle layer, which is the outermost layer of the hair follicle. When the cuticle is smooth it reflects the most light. An open or damaged cuticle should be repaired through conditioning treatments before it can receive and achieve exceptional color.

Changing your color is an exciting experience. But let's face it, it can also be a nerve-wracking one that may reap horrendous results. This is why I cannot stress enough the importance of putting color in the hands of a professional, not your neighbor or best friend.

A certified colorist can create new colors, enhance existing tones, and tone down unwanted color. Who knows what can happen when you color your hair at home and don't get the color you expected? Often the name on the box of an over-the-counter color is the brand name. Your colorist can match and/or enhance any and all colors and also add dimension (highlights, lowlights, tipping, and beliage techniques).

Start with a color consultation. During this session you and your colorist should share ideas. Bring photographs of the shades you're hoping to achieve. Choose swatches to visualize the color you would like. Get on the same page. Your colorist should take into consideration your skin tone, your desired color, and your natural color, and should record all of your previous color services. He or she should devise a plan of action as well as short- and long-term goals for your color journey.

Natural hair consists of more than one color. It is in fact several colors combined. Hair coloring is simply adding color to color or tone on tone. Colorists often talk about hues and tones when deciding on a color for their clients. Clarifying these concepts with you will help you to understand exactly what your colorist is talking about, and clarity is essential when it comes to changing your hair

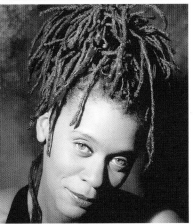

ADDING COLOR GIVES YOUR LOCS A NEW DIMENSION

BLONDE REMAINS EVER POPULAR WITH BOLD, TREND-SETTING WOMEN OF COLOR. POP STAR BEYONCÉ

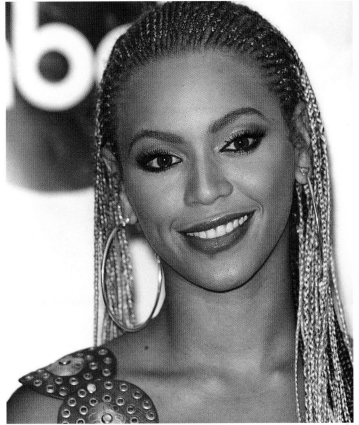

color. Hues are the colors the colorist can blend. Usually tone relates to your skin, but is often used to describe colors as warm or cool. Take a look at the chart below.

Color can have either a warm or cool intensity or tone. Warm tones are oranges, reds, and yellows. Blonde remains ever popular with bold, trend-setting women of color. Both Mary J. Blige and T-Boz of TLC are often credited with repopularizing this amazing color in the 90s. This millennium, think of the fashionable rapper Eve, the self-proclaimed "blonde bombshell," vocalist extraordinaire Cassandra Wilson, pop star Beyoncé, and the powerful percussionist Cindy Blackman.

Lovely browns have been worn by the entertainment icon Janet Jackson, the timeless jazz singer Dianne Reeves, as well as actress Jada Pinkett

The Color Process	The Color Properties	The Color Cautions
Rinse or color conditioners	Lasts 1 to 2 washings. Can be used for a test run before you apply more permanent color. Improves sheen and condition.	May stain clothes when hair is wet.
Semi-permanent opaque	Lasts 8 to 10 washings. Adds sheen and enhances the condition of the hair.	Prolonged use of dark colors may permanently darken hair. No dryer use with relaxed hair.
Demi-permanent	Lasts up to 2 months. Low peroxide.	When used the same day as relaxer, will lift hair color 2 to 3 levels.
Sheer glossings	Peroxide free. Moderate gray coverage. High gloss. Conditioning.	Virtually nothing. Recommended for relaxed hair. Hard to see on tightly coiled hair.
Tone on tone	Lasts permanently on hair shaft. New growth must be retouched every 3 to 4 weeks. Provides lift (if you want a change from black to blonde shades). Great for short, natural, and relaxed styles.	Breakage may occur if deep conditioners are not used. Look for low ammonia contents.
Double process	Touch up in 3 weeks. Lifts color. Various shades of color can be applied.	Works best on straight, wavy, or natural hair. Not recommended for relaxed styles.
Bleach/Ultra blondes	Touch up in 3 weeks. Lifts color up to platinum.	Recommended for natural and short hair. Always condition.
Highlights (Tipping and Beliage)	Touch up in 3 months. Creates blocks of color. Adds dimension.	Recommended for all textures as well as relaxed hair. Always condition.
Lowlights	Creates blocks of color. Tones highlights.	Recommended for toning highlights on any texture.

Smith, who has looked great wearing practically every color on the spectrum from jet black to platinum blonde. We've seen the strong presence of all shades of red and mahogany for the past three years, yet it still has incredible staying power. The gospel-singing sister group Mary Mary and Destiny's Child member Kelly Rowland have looked fantastic in this cherry color.

Cool tones are blue violets and greens. The R&B newcomer Ashanti always looks great with her black tresses whether she wears them straight or wavy, as do actresses Gabrielle Union and Garcelle Beauvais-Nilon.

Warm tones tend to brighten or lighten your aura while cool tones tend to darken or subdue your aura. The aura that I speak of is that inner glow that we are born with. You know that glow that a baby or a pregnant woman has or the glow from a fresh tan? Well that's exactly what color can do for you. Color will bring out the natural aura that we all have.

The majority of women of color tend to have darker hair. Lightening the hair to levels above level five, which is a medium brown, will result in red or orange tones. Many times red and orange tones will appear regardless of which color product you use.

Color challenges. Pregnancy and white hair often require a special approach when coloring. As I explained in Chapter 2, Healthy Hair Is Happy Hair, pregnant women should generally stay away from color while they are pregnant, especially in the first trimester. If you are presently coloring with a permanent color, why not try a semi- or demi-color closer to your natural color while pregnant, and then go back to full color services after the child is born. This is a safer alternative for both you and your child. Granted, there are women who have told me that they have colored their hair during their pregnancy and everything was fine. In good faith I feel obliged to give you all the facts. The choice is ultimately yours, of course.

Color Level Sidebar

Level 1 = Black
Level 2 = Darkest Brown
Level 3 = Dark Brown
Level 4 = Medium Brown
Level 5 = Light Brown
Level 6 = Dark Blonde
Level 7 = Medium Blonde
Level 8 = Light Blonde
Level 9 = Very Light Blonde
Level 10 = Lightest Blonde
Levels 11 and/or 12 = Ultra Blonde*

*I always use Ultra Blonde series to achieve a very light blonde without bleaching.

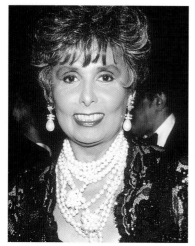

Glorious Grays. Silver or white hair is beautiful in and of itself. There are specific glosses and shampoos that can enhance your silver hair to keep the hair shining while eliminating that yellow cast that silver hair is susceptible to. Clairol Shimmer Lights Shampoo is excellent, as well as Goldwell Definition Pearl Condtioner or Color Enhancer. Stick with semi- or demi-permanents such as deep mahoganies, reds, and browns for highlighting silver hair. Ask your colorist for her recommendation. For those of you who want to color silver hair, natural highlights and a demi-permanent color will enhance your hair with wonderful tones.

LENA HORNE PERSONIFIES CLASS AND SOPHISTICATION WITH HER GREAT-LOOKING SILVER HAIR

COLORING TIPS

1. Ask your colorist if she or he is certified and with what company. Most stylists can successfully apply semi-permanents and color. However for special techniques, dimensional coloring, and color correction, always seek a certified colorist.

2. Semi-permanents last longer when applied after the conditioning treatment. Red roots/hot roots can be avoided by making sure your stylist applies your color to the base (the ¼ inch of hair closest to the scalp) last.

3. A healthy, conditioned head of hair is the key to maintaining long-lasting color.

4. Color conditioners really do preserve the freshly applied color, especially in the summer and in the sun. Use them. Try Aveda Color Conditioners or Biolage Earth Tone Color Reserve or Goldwell Definition Color Conditioners.

5. Permanent color should receive touch ups at least every four weeks for consistency.

6. Use shampoos and conditioners specially formulated for colored hair. Both will enhance the hair color. Try Aveda Color Reserve System or Textures and Tones System.

Hair is an extension of your thoughts and your thoughts are like pearls. Therefore, your hairs are pearls. They have to be protected and nurtured. And every hair shall be counted. —Lauryn Hill

Celebrity Memoir of
LAURYN HILL

Several years ago, five-time Grammy Award winner Lauryn Hill asked me to assist her in creating a brand-new look for the cover of the Fugees' album *The Score*. She desperately desired a different color for her naturally dark brown hair. At the time Lauryn was studying at Columbia University while simultaneously recording the debut album. Needless to say, her time was limited.

Lauryn's initial concerns were regarding the long- and short-term effects of coloring her hair. What would the color do to her hair? Would it dry out her hair? How long would it last? What were the repercussions of bleaching her hair? Was this a double process or just a tint? And most important, could she go back to her original color and if so, how soon?

I sensed Lauryn's apprehension and suggested we discuss the process step by step. Once I answered each one of her questions thoroughly, she relaxed and expressed with certainty that she trusted me to handle the magical transformation.

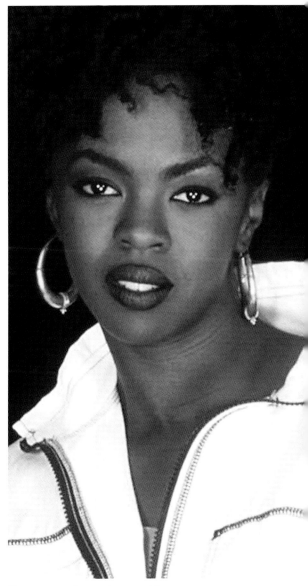

RECORDING ARTIST LAURYN HILL

With soothing music playing in the background, I blended the formula, then proceeded to apply the mixture to her hair. It was necessary to first alter the color of Lauryn's natural hair while preparing the hair to receive the new red-hued tone.

Hair that is very black usually requires a few sessions to achieve the proper color, especially when lifting black tint from any textured hair. Natural hair is one texture that can take on a little more imagination of color. However, I wouldn't recommend it for chemically relaxed hair.

The procedure was actually quite simple—decolorize, tint, and condition, condition, condition. I used one of my favorite professional color product lines, Logics decolorizer gel and Logics crème colors. They work fabulously on textured hair.

Lauryn was completely shocked after the first session. Her hair was reddish-orange. She wanted a light brown without too much red and I explained to her the process would require two more sessions. I needed one more decolorizing session and then we could add the precise color.

Clients must be certain that they truly desire the new color for a lengthy period of time or at least be willing to cut their hair in a short style, particularly if they want to try new colors. Lauryn was very determined to achieve her custom color and opted to sport a wide variety of hats until the entire process was completed.

The final result was a radiant Lauryn with a beautiful new color. Eventually she went back to the black locs, and eventually she cut off her locs. A few years later, I styled her cropped natural free hair for the July 2002 issue of *Essence*. She'd been cutting her hair herself, and requested that I style her hair at the shoot.

When we met in March 2002 for the July *Essence* cover shoot, Lauryn stated that it was a new day for her and she was not the same person she used to be. Things had changed and she was no longer conforming to what people would like her to be and how they would like to see her. At a performance at Jones Beach that summer, she wore her hair in a short 'fro, with only a hint of makeup, and glamorous dangling earrings. She had a different life. She had her children to think about. She still loved her hair, makeup, and style, but she now chose a different approach—simple and less dramatic.

One of the great rewards of textured hair is the ability to start anew!

Celebrity Memoir of
DEE DEE BRIDGEWATER

Dee Dee Bridgewater is a Paris-based jazz vocalist diva signed to Verve Records. She's also a theatrical performer, Grammy Award–winning singer, mother, wife, and artist whose infectious spirit soars. She first came to visit me at Dyaspora Salon in the spring of 2000. She whisked through wearing an Isaac Mizrahi ensemble, speaking fluent French on her cell phone. Absolutely exquisite. We quickly decided on color and wraps for her newly started locs. I colored and wrapped her locs and off she went in her limo.

JAZZ VOCALIST
DEE DEE BRIDGEWATER

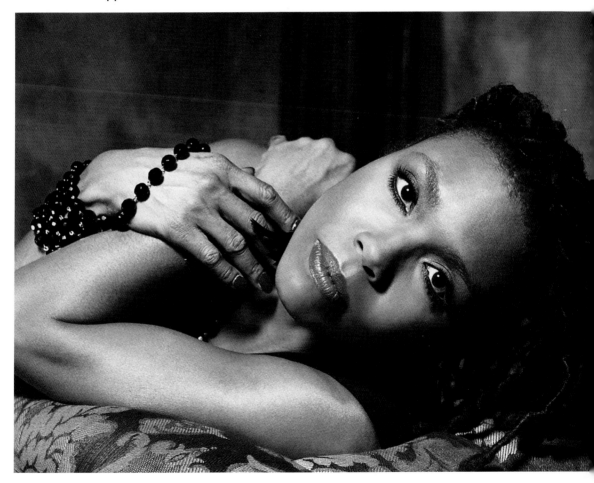

In November 2001, Dee Dee called me to sculpt her hair for the cover of her new CD. Dee Dee wanted more color after seeing another jazz vocalist client of mine, Lenora Zenzalia-Helm, at a performance in New York City. She wanted the same multi-colored highlights on her locs.

I spoke in depth with Michaela Angela Davis, the stylist for the shoot and the fashion director at *Honey* magazine, about the look and feel they wanted. They wanted to lighten Dee Dee's hair, but I advised against it. We decided we would keep her dark brown color and highlight with colored natural hair wraps, which would ultimately be healthier for her hair.

I colored her hair a dark brown and wrapped her locs with afro hair in the same color to make her locs stronger. We were pressed for time, so I made red loc extensions and placed them in Dee Dee's hair instead of wrapping all of her hair, which would have taken hours. I created a new method to instantly obtain color highlights without hairpins or combs. They can be taken out easily and effortlessly. When I showed Dee Dee what was going in her hair she told me I was a wizard. I placed the pieces in her hair and styled her for the first photo in about 20 minutes. I worked diligently and knocked it out just like that. The results were terrific—a full head of beautifully highlighted loc extensions, intertwined in twists cascading down the side of her face. Whew!

FIFTEEN

Cover Shots

cannot emphasize enough what a blessing it is to make a living at what I love doing. It is also a privilege to have my artistry recognized and appreciated by others. Quite a few times that recognition has led to a highly coveted magazine or CD cover.

Working with musicians and models to convey a look that will entice you, the reader or listener, yet satisfy me, the artist, and please the editor and record label is hard work, to say the least. More important though, it is incredibly rewarding. It is someone else saying, "I trust your vision and creative abilities. I like your talent." And that sounds good coming from any client, whether they are a nine-to-fiver or the latest pop star. As a matter of fact, all my clients are celebrities to me—each one in their own unique way has helped me to celebrate life.

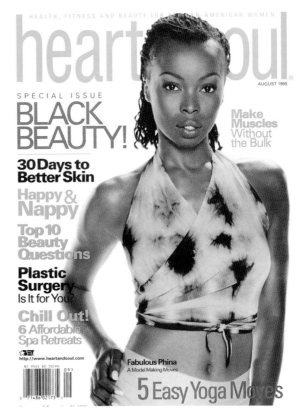

Heart & Soul MAGAZINE

THIS WAS MY FIRST COVER FOR *HEART & SOUL* WITH THE MODEL AND FINE ARTIST PHINA OKHURA, PHOTOGRAPHED BY MARC BAPTISTE. HER LOCS WERE REALLY HEALTHY AND IN GREAT CONDITION, SO THEY WERE VERY EASY TO WORK WITH. PHINA HAS A BEAUTIFUL SPIRIT AND BOTH HER HAIR AND SKIN REFLECTED THAT.

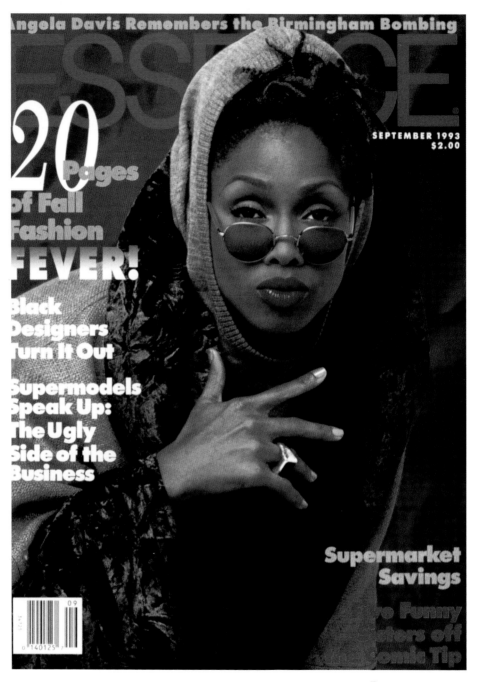

THIS WAS MY FIRST *ESSENCE* COVER. I STYLED THE MODEL'S LOCS BY ACTUALLY CUTTING A FEW OF MY OWN GOLDEN LOCS AND ADDING THEM TO HER HAIR FOR ENHANCED COLOR. IRONICALLY, SHE WORE A HAT, AS DID LAURYN HILL IN MY SECOND *ESSENCE* MAGAZINE COVER.

SIXTEEN

Improvisation

Glamorous Styles for Men and Women

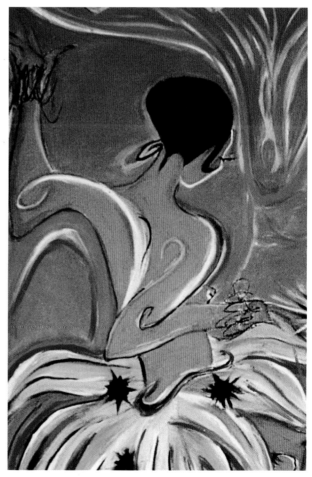

There are thousands of hair stylists across the country, but not all of them are true visionaries. Hair artistry is the epitome of free expression. I wanted to share with you the exotic creations of other stylists as well as my own. These exciting textured looks may not be meant for everyday wear but they offer a glimpse of avant garde, creative, free hair styling. Each one of the hairstylists featured is not only highly respected, but incredibly talented. They've created gorgeous styles on a variety of hair textures.

Some say life imitates art. Others say art imitates life. Even more say imitation is the greatest form of flattery. I say go ahead, imitate, duplicate, and create with your textured hair.

RENALDO'S JOSEPHINE BAKER

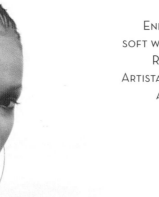

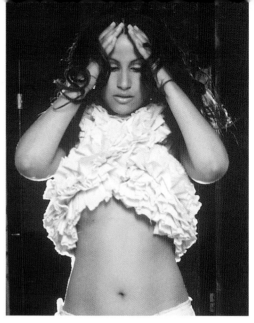

DESIGNER BRAIDS BY KHAMIT KINKS

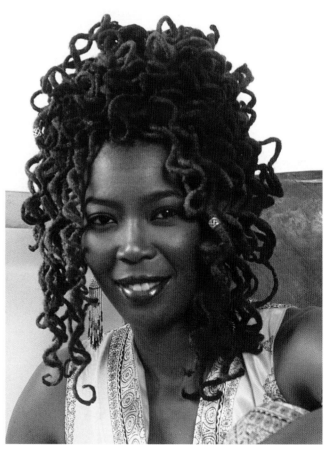

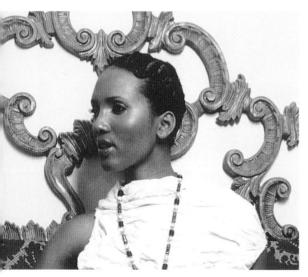

SOFT FINGER WAVES BY DIANE DA COSTA

THE SWIRLY CULTIVATED LOCS BY ONA THE
LOCKSMYTH, OF LOCKSMYTHS HAIR GROOMERS

Let loose, let go, and have fun! May the artwork in this chapter serve as inspiration for you to realize your textured hair has boundless potential.

What better way to convey the newness, the forward movement of naturally textured hair and styles than to gather some of the finest young jazz musicians in the world at the Akwaaba Mansion, a bed and breakfast, and Akwaaba Café (a Moshan enterprise). Monique Greenwood, the former editor-in-chief of *Essence*, and her husband, Glenn, own both establishments in the Stuyvesant Heights section of Brooklyn, New York.

Jazz today is often viewed as conservative or as music appreciated by the "conservative crowd." Unfortunately, in some circles it's even seen as a dying art. Yet in actuality, jazz is still leading the way, showing the world that everything old is new again whether retro or vintage is "in" or "out." Jazz is current. Jazz is relevant. Jazz is free style. Jazz is improv. And so is textured hair. So why not dress up our jazz musicians and do up their hair to show the world that some of today's top jazz performers' forward thinking and forward movement is reflected in their hair.

Wouldn't you know it? On the day of the shoot, the patrons of Akwaaba Café were treated to an impromptu performance by

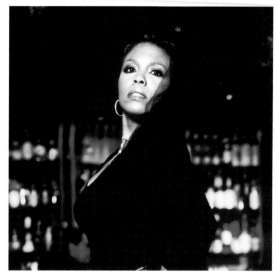

DEE DEE BRIDGEWATER, WITH CONTESSA UPDO LOCS
(*photographed by Mark Higashino*)

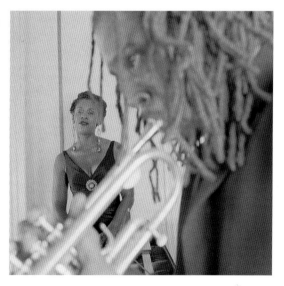

TRUMPETER ROY HARGROVE WITH LOOSE LOCS AND VOCALIST LENORA ZENZALIA-HELM WITH LOCS UPDO
(*photographed by Niya Bascom*)

the Grammy Award–winning jazz trumpeter Roy Hargrove (a jazz veteran who spends more time touring out of the country than in). It didn't matter that it wasn't scheduled, wasn't part of the plans. He just went with his feelings, his spirit—much like his hair and the hair of the other musicians here: free, moving, and full of energy.

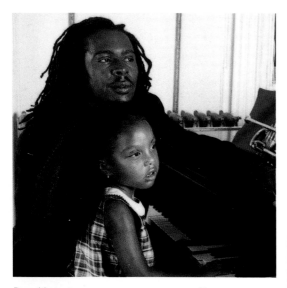

ROY HARGROVE WITH HIS DAUGHTER, KAMALA, WITH NATURAL, FREE HAIR *(photographed by Niya Bascom)*

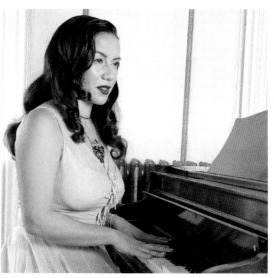

BRAZILIAN VOCALIST CLAUDIA ACUNA WITH SOFT WAVES *(photographed by Niya Bascom)*

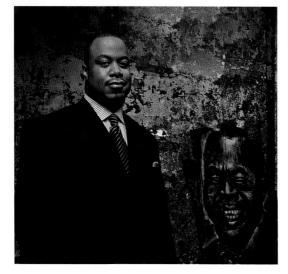

NICHOLAS PAYTON TRIBUTE TO LOUIS ARMSTRONG CD. NICHOLAS IS A SWEET, QUIET, AND HUMBLE GENTLEMAN. GROOMED WITH LIGHT MAKEUP AND A SHORT CAESAR HAIRCUT, HE WAS READY TO GO. THIS WAS A FUN AND PLAYFUL DAY WITH THE GREAT JAZZ TRUMPETER. HOLLIS KING, THE MAD HATTER/V.P./CREATIVE DIRECTOR OF VERVE RECORDS, CREATED THE MOOD AND ORCHESTRATED THE SHOOT.

Salon Directory

Natural/Textured Hair*

UNITED STATES

Alabama

Artistic Braids & Naturals
3102 Greensboro Ave., Suite 5A
Tuscaloosa, AL 35401
(205) 342-3085

California

Hair Today Hair Tomorrow
308 40th Street
Oakland, CA 94609
(510) 654-0392

I.F.B.A.—Institute of Fine
    Braidery Arts
4329 Degnan Blvd.
Los Angeles, CA 90008
(323) 299-8994

Oh! My Nappy Hair
805 South La Brea Avenue
Los Angeles, CA 90036
(323) 939-3999

Nadira Belcher, Loctician
email: nadiloc@aol.com

Colorado

Rumors Beauty Salon and
    Barber Shop
2350 S. Chambers Road,
    Unit B
Aurora, CO 80014
(720) 748-1400
*Specializing in twist, braids,
weaves, and everything else
concerning hair.*

* Partial natural salon listing provided by: napptural.com

Connecticut

Mahogany's Natural Hair
   Heaven
122 Read Street
New Haven, CT 06511
(203) 776-7975

Florida

Mandisa Ngozi Braiding Gallery
1313 N. Gadsden Street
Tallahassee, FL 32303
(850) 561-0330
www.mandisa-ngozi.com

Natural Trend Setters
5100 West Commercial
   Boulevard
Tamarac, FL 33319
(954) 486-1414

Skies Limited Braiding Salon
2027 S. Adams Street
Tallahassee, FL 32301
(850) 222-4421
*This salon also sells beauty
supplies. The salon is located
within walking distance of
Florida A&M University
(FAMU).*

Georgia

Braids, Weaves & Things
1180 Ralph D. Abernathy Blvd.
Atlanta, GA 30310
(404) 753-4555

Deeply Rooted @ Your Majesty
   Beauty & Barber Salon
2327 Austell Road
Marietta, GA 30060
(770) 434-1411

Khamit Kinks
792 North Highland Avenue,
   Suite 1B
Atlanta, GA 30306
(404) 607-9805

Illinois

Ajes Salon
648 W. Randolph Street
Chicago, IL 60661
(312) 454-1133

Amazon Salon
1900 South Clark Street,
   Suite 103
Chicago, IL 60616
(312) 674-9033

Braids Designer
14524 Kimbark Avenue
Dolton, IL 60419
(708) 849-2475
*Braids, natural dreadlocks,
and dreadlock extensions*

Why Knot
851 W. Randolph Street
Chicago, IL 60607
(312) 421-6580

Indiana

Swing Tyme Total Salon &
   Day Spa
2441 E. 65th Street
Indianapolis, IN 46220
Salon (317) 251-5604
Message Center (317) 465-8581
Fax (317) 251-5154
www.thierrybaptiste.com

Louisiana

Nature's Crown
111 East Airport Avenue
Baton Rouge, LA 70806
(225) 218-8035
*Braids, locs, interlocking, twists,
weaves and sisterlocks*

Maryland

Twist Hair Salon
7104 Minstrel Way, Suite A
Columbia, MD 21045
(410) 381-3700

Thomascine Smith
Last Stop Hair Shop
2890 Hillen Road
Baltimore, MD 21218
(410) 243-3133

Michigan

Everettes Corn-Rows & Braiding
   Academy
16038 E. 8 Mile Road
Detroit, MI 48205
1-800-CORNROW or
   (313) 527-2884

Mane Taming Hair Salon
21645 W. 8 Mile Road
Detroit, MI 48219
(313) 255-8650

Missouri

Cuts of Class II
Goodfellow Blvd. &
Interstate 70
St. Louis, MO 63120

Coloring, braiding, locs, twists,
and natural hairstyles; ask for
Starr

Napps
6267 Delmar Blvd.
St. Louis, MO 63130
(314) 727-0312

New Jersey

Afrakuts
8 Cleveland Street
Orange, NJ 07050
(973) 672-2887

Braids R Us
301 Irvington Avenue
South Orange, NJ 07079
(973) 761-6737
Braiding, two-strand twists, locs
and locs maintenance

Native Essence
1408 Springfield Avenue
Irvington, NJ 07111
(973) 375-2080

New York

Upstate
Blues Bros. Barber Shop
441 Hawley Avenue

Syracuse, NY 13203
(315) 472-0398

New York City
Afrigenix
220 West 72nd Street
New York, NY 10023
(212) 873-0688
Weaves and braids

Beautopia Lifestyle Salon
Aveda Concept
4357 White Plains Road
Bronx, NY 10466
(718) 994-5716

Curve Salon
(Brooklyn location;
   by appointment only)
(718) 852-2600
www.curve-salon.com

Khamit Kinks
4 Leonard Street
New York, NY 10013
(212) 965-9100

Jelani Hair Salon
54 West 39th Street
New York, NY 10018
(212) 265-7206

Locks 'N' Chops Natural Hair
   Salons
365 West 34th Street
New York, NY 10001
(212) 244-2306

Locksmyths African Loc
   Groomers
214 Greene Avenue
Brooklyn, NY 11238
(718) 855-3243
email: Locksmyths@hotmail.com

Mishon Mishon
Natural Hair Care Artist
1015 Fulton St. (bet. Grand
   and Downing)
Brooklyn, NY 11238
(718) 636-1660

Red Creative Art Salon
104 Bainbridge Street
Brooklyn, NY 11233
(718) 221-5581

Derrick Scurry
www.derrickscurry.com
Natural hair specialist

Soween by Ngone Sow Inc.
466 Nostrand Avenue

Brooklyn, NY 11216
(718) 789-2655

Turning Heads Salon
218 Lenox Avenue
New York, NY 10027
(212) 828-4600

Tendrils
475 Myrtle Avenue
Brooklyn, NY 11205
(718) 875-3811

Hair Talk
85-15 Main Street, Suite E
Jamaica, NY 11435
(718) 526-3663

North Carolina

Braids 'R Beautiful
201-3 S. Brightleaf Blvd.
Smithfield, NC 27577
(919) 934-0009

Glory Locs
2240 Grey Fox Lane
Winston-Salem, NC 27106
email: Ahardinv@msn.com
(336) 922-0723, (336) 971-7219
Starting and maintaining locs

Pennsylvania

Au Naturale
6755 Germantown Avenue
Philadelphia, PA 19119
(215) 848-7848
fax (215) 991-6762
email: info@aunaturalehair.com
www.aunaturalehair.com
Specializing in two-strand twists, coils, starter locs, loc styling, herbal hair color, loc maintenance, two-strand twists with extensions, micros, synthetic braids, and intricate natural hair cornrows.

Endless Creations
271 South 44th Street
Philadelphia, PA 19104
(215) 662-1753
Offers classes on how to start, maintain, and retighten sisterlocks.

South Carolina

Inner Image Salon
36 Blake Street
Charleston, SC 29403
(843) 577-0136

Texas

Ebony Hair Expressions
5105 San Jacinto Street
Houston, TX 77004
(713) 520-1283

Soul Scissors
4400 Almeda Road
Houston, TX 77004
(713) 739-7685

Virginia

B.A.D.—Braids & Dreds, Inc.
121 Wyck Street, Suite 209
Richmond, VA 23225
(804) 276-3200
www.braid-designer.com
Specializing in—loc maintenance, starting locs, interlocking and undetectable cornrows. We offer total and complete **FREE** *maintenance every two weeks for the life of your braid style.*

Essence of Braid & Weaving
321A Brook Road
Richmond, VA 23220
(804) 643-5420

Washington

Gorgeous Braids
2301 South Jackson Street
Seattle, WA 98144
(206) 720-0349

Melinda's Micro's
66 Tacoma Mall Blvd.
Tacoma, WA 98409
(253) 473-1452
www.nebsnow.com/
    melindasmicros
email: Bradleymissmoe@aol.com
*Providing professional braiding
services for women and children.
Specializing in micro-braiding,
silky dreads, and more.*

District of Columbia

Cornrows & Company
5401 14th Street, N.W.
Washington, DC 20015
(202) 723-1827

Oliver Natural Hair Salon
5225 Connecticut Avenue,
    N.W., #210
Washington, DC 20015
(202) 686-9714
Fax: (202) 686-9715
www.oliveraromatics.com

SisTwist—The Stress Free Zone
2816 Georgia Avenue, N.W.
Washington, DC 20001
(202) 299-9013
www.sistwist.com
From perm to natural

Twist-N-Turns Natural Hair
7416 George Avenue, N.W.,
    Suite 102
Washington, DC 20012
(202) 882-2309

U.S. Virgin Islands

Sera's Beauty Supply/Salon
1AH Estate Diamond
Christiansted, U.S. Virgin Islands
    00851
(340) 778-1000

INTERNATIONAL SALONS
Canada

Abantu Beauty Salon
on Kingsway
Burnaby, BC V5H 2BC
(604) 431-4589
*Clara Amaguru was named the
World's Best Braider at the 2000
World Natural Hair & Beauty
Show.*

Michael's on Main
Main Street
Chilliwack, BC
(604) 792-6161
Specializing in braids

Germany

Magic Style Haarflecht-Atelier
Daimlerstr. 75, 74211
  Heilbronn/Leingarten
Telefon: 07131/576860
Mobil: 0177/6585641
Fax: 07131/401697
email: MagicStyle@AddCom.de
Web: http://go.to/MagicStyle
*Braids, cornrows, dreadlocks, hair
extensions*

Holland (Netherlands)

Hair Police of Amsterdam
113 Kerkstraat
Amsterdam

United Kingdom

Back to Eden
Natural Hair and Scalp Clinic
14 Westmoreland Road
(off Walworth Road)
Walworth, London SE17 2AY
44 207 703 3173

Bold and Natural
200 High Road
Leytonstone
London E11 3HU
44 20 8221 0524
*Steam treatments, comb twist,
two-strand twist, flat twist, spiral
twist, silky dreads, start and
maintain locs*

Streetsahead
112c Brixton Hill
London SW2 1AH
0208 671 3357 *(Contact June)*
*They use a wide range of natural
herbal hair products. They also
have a video that helps parents of
mixed-race children manage
their hair.*

Salons offering other services

UNITED STATES
California

Eclipse
7250 Melrose Avenue
Los Angeles, CA 90046

Umberto Salon
Janet Zeitoun

416 N. Canon Drive
Beverly Hills, CA 90210
(310) 274-6395

Jordan's Salon
Rhonda Smith
409 N. Robertson Blvd.
West Hollywood, CA 90048
(310) 288-0874

Sean Smith
Ashby's Coiffures
722 S. La Brea Avenue
Los Angeles, CA 90036
(323) 938-9151
(310) 877-2514 (cell)

Sessions Salon
761 E. Green Street
Pasadena, CA 91101
(626) 795-8856
Nekko/The Christal Agency

Florida

Le Boe European Spa
9108 Wiles Road
Coral Springs, FL 33067
(954) 755-1744
www.Leboedayspa.com
*Specializing in glamour updos
and specialty braiding*

Georgia

Van Michael Salons
39 West Paces Perry Road
Atlanta, GA 30305
(404) 237-4664

Illinois

It's Only Hair
25 East Washington Street
Chicago, IL 60602
(312) 853-1105

Marianne Strokirk Salon
316 West Chesnut Street
Chicago, IL 60610
Francis Gillespie
(312) 944-4428 x210

Massachusetts

Olive Benson Salon
565 Columbus Avenue
Boston, MA 02118
(617) 247-3333

New York

John Atchison
39 W. 56th Street
New York, NY 10019
(212) 265-7206
Precision cuts

Antonio Prieto
25 W. 19th Street
New York, NY 10011
(212) 255-3741
Color/cuts

Artista Salon
139 Fifth Avenue, 2nd fl.
New York, NY 10011
www.artistaspa.com
Color/cuts

Brittanica & Associates
864 Lexington Avenue
New York, NY 10021
(212) 879-7030
Relaxer/cut/weaves

Benisty Salon
152 West 26th Street
New York, NY 10001
(646) 336-6231
Color/cuts

DL.d Reps—
    Beauty.Style.Design.
Diane Da Costa
244 Fifth Avenue, Suite 2231
New York, NY 10001
(212) 252-4472
*Image consultant, color
specialist, and bridal hair and
makeup*

Darryl Bennett
Picasso Salon
257 W. 34th St., 2nd fl.
New York, NY 10001
(212) 760-0909
www.dbennett.com

Expectations & Innovations
    Diane Nurse
179 Madison Avenue
New York, NY 10016
(212) 696-2420
Relaxers/cut/style

Edgehill Beauty Boutique
143 West 22nd Street
New York, NY 10011
(212) 243-7200
Weaves and cuts

Edris Salon
430 West 14th Street, 3rd fl.
New York, NY 10014
(212) 989-6800
Color/cut/style

Felipe
Helio DeSouza
1107 Second Avenue
New York, NY 10022
(212) 223-8731
Precision cuts

Follicles
709 Fulton Street
Brooklyn, NY 11217
(718) 522-0557

Gallant Salon
14 W. 55th Street
New York, NY 10019
(212) 246-3471

Hair Fashions East
411 Park Avenue South
New York, NY 10016
(212) 686-7524
*Relaxers/cuts—hair care
specialists*

Le Chameleon
326 7th Avenue
Brooklyn, NY 11215
(718) 788-1700

Lush/Luxe Studios
385 Canal Street
New York, NY 10013
(917) 237-2051
Relaxer/color/cuts/weaves

LaVar Hair Designs
127 W. 72nd Street
New York, NY 10023
(212) 724-4492
Weaves and braids

Mo' Hair
244 East 13th Street
New York, NY 10003
(212) 533-8610

Owen Sandy Hair Design
265 West 23rd Street
New York, NY 10011
(212) 396-2747
Precision cuts

Sam Wong
296 Elizabeth Street
New York, NY 10012
(SoHo/NoHo/Little Italy)
(212) 219-9833
www.samwonghair.com

Patric Wellington
Salon Celeste
255 W. 23rd Street
New York, NY 10011
(212) 243-9379
Relaxer/precision cuts

Santa Cruz
66 Madison Avenue
New York, NY 10016
(212) 684-2386
Specializing in curly hair

Scott J. Salon & Spa
Aveda Concept Salon

257 Columbus Avenue
New York, NY 10023
(212) 769-0107
Color/cut—spa services

Styles Salon
5 W. 46th Street
New York, NY 10036
(212) 730-6340

Textures Salon
134 W. 26th St., 10th fl.
New York, NY 10001
(212) 243-1046

Studio One Hair Salon
Hadiiya Barbel
Brooklyn, NY 11208
www.hadiiyabarbel.com
Weaves/styling

Time Salon
9 Green Avenue
Brooklyn, NY 11238
(718) 522-9030

Texas

Emages Hair, USA
619 Richmond Avenue
Houston, Texas 77006
(713) 521-1420

District of Columbia

Zianni International Studios
1825 18th Street, N.W.
Washington, DC 20009
(202) 797-7706

INTERNATIONAL
Canada

Jazma Salon
136 Yorkville Avenue
Toronto, Ontario M5R 1C2
(416) 928-1888

Recommended
Products

Aveda—1-866-823-1425 (Aveda Concept Salons and Boutique Stores)
www.aveda.com

Carol's Daughter—Showroom—One South Elliot Place, Brooklyn, NY
11217, (718) 596-1862; toll-free phone orders, (877) 540-2101

Clinique—sold at Bloomingdale's, Saks Fifth Avenue, and Macy's

Gentle Treatment—sold at Target, Wal-Mart, and drug stores

Goldwell Color System—provided by professional colorists/
salons—www.goldwell.com

Kiehl's—Barneys, NYC, and The Flagship Store—109 3rd Avenue, NYC,
(212) 677-3171

KeraCare Products—Avlon/Affirm 1-800-332-8566 (sold in beauty
salons and beauty supply stores), www.avlon.com

Kérastase shampoo and conditioners—sold at upscale and select beauty
salons and beauty supply stores—www.kerastase.com

L'Oréal Majarel Professional Colors and Salons—www.Loreal.com

Optimum MultiMineral Relaxers—SoftSheen•Carson/L'Oréal,
www.lorealusa.com/prodbrand or www.softsheen-carson.com

Pantene Pro-V Shampoos and Conditioners—sold at Rite Aid, CVS,
and other drug stores

Neutrogena Shampoos and Conditioners—sold at Rite Aid, CVS, and
other drug stores

Matrix: Biolage Earth Tones Color Refreshing Conditioners—sold at your local hair salon or www.matrix.com

Mizani Relaxer System, Shampoos, Conditioners, and Finishing Products—1-800-342-7661; call for a certified Mizani Salon near you

Paul Mitchell Tea Tree Special Shampoo and Conditioner—www.paulmitchell.com

Phytologie/Phytospecific—sold at Barneys

References

Aveda Corporation, Estée Lauder. Indigenous ingredients.

Bundles, A'lelia. *On Her Own Ground: The Life and Times of Madam C. J. Walker*. New York: Scribner/Simon & Schuster, 2001.

Colomer International. *Voilà Color Manual*. New York: Revlon Professional.

Cook-Bolden, Dr. Fran, dermatologist: Interview on scalp disorders, NYC.

Evans, Nekhena. *Hairlocking: Everything You Need to Know: African, Dread and Nubian*. New York: A & B Publishers Group, 1999.

hooks, bell. *Sisters of the Yam: Black Women and Self-Recovery*. Boston: South End Press, 1993.

Kimura, Margaret. *Asian Beauty*. New York: Harper Resource, 2001.

Kinard, Tulani. *No Lye*. New York: St. Martin's Press, 1997.

Kofi, Alvin (Bushmen USA): Interview on Samburu people of Masai Tribe, London.

Locks, 3rd ed. New York: A & B Books, 1991.

Matrix, International: Biolage Earth Tone color chart.

McCurtis, Dr. Henry: Interview on stress management, NYC.

Pirello, Christina. *Glow: A Prescription for Radiant Health and Beauty*. New York: Penguin Putnam, 2001.

Salon Fundamentals: A Resource for Your Cosmetology Career. Chicago: Pivot Point International, 2000.

Simmons, Dr. Deborah, dermatologist: Interview on disorders of the scalp, NYC.

Walsh, Neale Donald. *Communion with God*. New York: Penguin Putnam, 2000.

Webster's Dictionary, American Edition. New York: Barnes & Noble, 1999.

Art Credits

Unless otherwise indicated, all interior photographs by George Larkins.

Foreword

p. xii—Blair Underwood/Kwaku Alston

Introduction

p. xvi—Diane Da Costa/Roberto Ligresti

p. xviii—Massai warrior illustration/Alvin Kofi/Bushmen USA (Tehuti Productions)

p. xx—Lauryn Hill/Anthony Cutajar, courtesy of London Features International

p. xxi—Kent Williams/Kevin Dickens, KD Studios, NYC

Appreciating the Beauty of Naturally Textured Hair

p. 6—Tweet/courtesy of Elektra Records

p. 7—Alicia Keys/Courtesy of J Records

pp. 10 and 11—Roshumba/Matthew Jordan Smith

Healthy Hair Is Happy Hair

p. 14—Cassandra Wilson/courtesy of Blue Note/EMI

Diane's Bag

p. 44—"Afro Love Sista," illustration by Renaldo Davidson, Renaldo
Davidson Art Studio Co., NYC/photo by George Larkins
p. 49—Hikari Shears/courtesy of Hikari, Inc.

In Harmony

p. 54—Dyaspora Salon/courtesy of Diane Da Costa

Shear Perfection

p. 62—Hikari Shears/courtesy of Hikari, Inc.
p. 64—Nicole Sterling/courtesy of Dekar Lawson

Chemically Speaking

p. 70—Stylist: Tina Person, Brittanica & Associates/Eric von Lockhart
p. 72—Author styling hair/courtesy of Dekar Lawson
p. 74—Alicia Hall/Jinsey Dauk for Jinsey.com
p. 74—Tracy Grant/Gregg Routt
p. 75—Tamia/courtesy of Elektra Entertainment

Part II Achieve It!

p. 80—Dee Dee Bridgewater/Mark Higashino, courtesy of Verve Records
p. 82—Blair Underwood/Kwaku Alston
p. 82—Braids/Gordon Christmas

Natural Sets & Styles

p. 84—Lenny Kravitz/London Features International, courtesy of Virgin Records

p. 84—Bantu knots model/Marc Baptiste

p. 84—Beverly Bond/John Peden

p. 89—Retro Bantu knots/Marc Baptiste

p. 90—Line illustration/James Walker

p. 91—Beverly Bond/John Peden

p. 95—Lenny Kravitz/London Features International, courtesy of Virgin Records

pp. 96, 97—Line illustrations/James Walker

Twists & Turns

p. 98—Janine Green/Matthew Jordan Smith

p. 105—Cindy Blackman/Jimmy Bruch, *Someday* CD, courtesy of Highnote Records

Coils & Curls

p. 110—Denise Kerr/Matthew Jordan Smith

p. 111—Janine Green retro photo/Peter Ogilvie Photography

p. 113—Blair Underwood/ Kwaku Alston

p. 115—Line illustrations/James Walker

Locking & Tightening Up

p. 116—Yami Bolo/Donna Ranieri, courtesy of Verve Records

p. 119—Coily locks/Matthew Jordan Smith

p. 122—Dee Dee Bridgewater/Mark Higashino, courtesy of Verve Records

p. 123—Retro locs/Matthew Jordan Smith

pp. 124 and 125—Line illustrations/James Walker

p. 126—Roy Hargrove/Jack Guy, courtesy of Verve Records

p. 128—Illustrations/James Walker

Braids & Weaves

p. 130—Nene N'diaye, stylist, Cherokee Braids, Khamit Kinks,
www.khamitkinks.com/George Larkins

p. 132—Tyra Banks/London Features International

p. 133—Alicia Keys/Courtesy of J Records

p. 134—Nene N'diaye, stylist, Cherokee Braids, Khamit Kinks,
www.khamitkinks.com/George Larkins

p. 135—Model with braids for Dyaspora Salon/Gordon Christmas

p. 137—Retro ponytails/George Larkins

p. 139—Weaves/Matthew Jordan Smith

The Aura of Color & Illumination

p. 151—Lenora Zenzalia-Helm/Preston Thomas, thevisualear.com

p. 151—Beyoncé/courtesy of London Features International

p. 154—Lena Horne/courtesy of London Features International

p. 155—Lauryn Hill/Anthony Cutajar, courtesy of London Features
International

p. 157—Dee Dee Bridgewater/Mark Higashino, courtesy of Verve
Records

Cover Shots

p. 159—Marc Baptiste/courtesy of *Heart & Soul* magazine, Vanguard
Media

p. 160—Marc Baptiste/courtesy of Essence Communications/
Partnership, Ltd.

Improvisation

Acknowledgments

Praise God and give him thanks for allowing me to bring forth my creativity. Through him all things are possible. My parents Naomi and Linval Da Costa—It is done—I Love You—thank you for letting my spirit pass through both of you. I'm a butterfly and I'm flying free.

My brothers and sisters—Heather, Sharon, Wee, Lisa, and Jamiel—who have all endured so much while I've taken time out to write this book, I hope it was worth the wait. Henry—We did it!!!!!!!

My God daughters: Deanna, Kamala, Noa, and also Ariel and Mya—you energize me and give me love—who inspire me to write my children's hair books. To Jordan and Julian, Marcus, Sicily, Toni, and Anissa, the Thomkins family, and all my nieces and nephews, cousins, aunts, and uncles—you know who you are—the tribe is too big to name.

Blair and Desiree Underwood and family for your continuing love and support. Kevin, Chrystal, and Curtis, you're the best.

Merlin Bobb—who inspired me to be the best hairstylist from the very beginning of my career. Thanks for the love and support.

My creative soul brother, Roy Hargrove, for the many years we've shared together on your hair and making the mane stay.

My Soul Sister, Midwife, and co-writer on this baby project (giving birth for two years), Paula, you've endured more than your share—but continue to walk in the light.

Todd Wilson, you have lifted me up time and time again and I will always love you for that.

To my Soul Mate—you're a guiding light—your strength, renaissance presence and your inspiration pushes me to strive to the next level—you are a cherished friend and leader—I respect you for your brilliance, your drive, and for being the vessel that God has chosen to send his message to me. Thanks for your love.

To all those who made this possible and participated in this project. My Editor, Task Master, and Spin Doctor, Cherise Davis, for signing me to Simon & Schuster and bringing this book to fruition. Ally Edelhertz Peltier, for all your assistance in bringing the team and Simon & Schuster together. Julie Castiglia Agency for believing in this project.

To all those who have graced their presence in my chair and on this project I thank you. Dee Dee Bridgewater, Mr. Ed Gordon and Taylor, Lauryn Hill and Rohan Marley, Jacob Underwood, Lenny Kravitz, Cindy Blackman, Nicholas Payton, Claudia Acuna, Lenora Zenzalia-Helm, Alicia Hall, Leon, Chelsea, and Kia Dorsey, Elizabeth Martin, Deidre Poe and Evan, Genny Kellam and Kara Fowler.

Nicole Moore (theHotness.com & Kalifly), it all started with a book and a couch to sleep on, thanks for the love, girl. Kym Norsworthy, Worth Inc. Public Relations, thanks for the PR at Dyaspora and your belief and encouragement that set me on my path to put the first words from pen to paper—it will always be cherished. To Carol CJ Green being there at the right time all the time—and delivering. I owe you a big one. Love ya.

For all those who went through the birthing process and who were there from the very beginning with Dyaspora—Selena Rogers and family, my spiritual parents Karen and Kowan, Qubanni Goodwyn, Denise Kerr, Tracy, Joe and Zoë Chamberlin, Pamela Greenidge, Alicia and Marc Hines, Peggy, Jon and Eric Berry, Cheryl, Kym and Aoka Christensen, Reggie Scott (you did ask), Barry Phillips, Allen Harvey, CPA, Allen Noel, CPA, Judith for all those catered events, Grace Ann, Ron and Mya Blake, Epperson.

To all my Clients at Dyaspora Salon and Turning Heads for making me the stylist I am today.

Darryl Bennett—Thanks for your spirit and presence—fellow Christian—for taking me out of the Wildness. Darlene (Vera Wang), you were right on time.

Essence magazine, Susan Taylor, Mikki Taylor, Sandra Martin—for all the wonderful hairstyling years, *Heart & Soul, Honey,* and Joicelyn Dingle for my first editorial position. Len Burnett of Vanguard Media, Diane Weathers *(Essence),* Melissa Lawrence, Michaela angela Davis and Mario *(Honey),* Bethann Hardison, Bethann Mgmt., Diana Actual Mgmt., Audra LVR, Carol CJ Green, Kirsten and Renee (Noelle Elaine PR), Josh Glick.

Renee Cox, Martin Booth, Kwaku Alston, Niya Bascom, Matthew Jordan Smith, Marc Baptiste, Barron Claiborne, Jon Peden, Peter Ogilvie, Renaldo, Alvin Koki, Verve Records—Hollis King: you are the man—for your madness, creative energy, and insight. Donna: there are not enough words to express my gratitude—thank you so much. Jai St. Laurent: thank you for getting all the artists together for me time and time again and the entire creative department at Verve.

Susan and Lela of Illusions, Soul Fixins, Robin Knuess Matrix—Emiliani, Barron Carr of JP Morgan Chase, Jamaica Tourist Board, Dekar Lawson of Dekar Salon, Artista Salon, Shanon Ayers of Turning Heads, Ona and Dena of the Locksmyths, Annu and Theifa of Khamit Kinks, Monroe and the *entire family* at Akwaaba Café, Monique Greenwood of Akwaaba Mansion, Latrice Verette, Jim and Gab of Platinum Investment Properties: Thanks for all you've done. Michael, Doreen, and all the stylists at Beautopia Lifestyle Salon: Thanks for keeping my hair done through this whole process. Tracy Sherrod Literary Services: God Bless You.

The Creative Crew: Thanks for your patience, support, and creative input—This project is a labor of love and could not have been accomplished without each and every one of you. God Bless.

My Hero: Madam C. J. Walker for her entrepreneurial spirit, and my hair designers and cosmetology mentors: Melvin Bridgewater, Owen Sandy, John Atchison, and Sam Wong—precision cutting, Ademola Mandela (Kinapps, Locs and Chops)—Master Barbering and Locking, Olive Benson—Styling, George Buckner, Felipe, Oscar James, and Derrick Scurry for your great quotes.

Matrix, Logics, and Aveda Color: you've made my life very colorful. Dekar Lawson for your freestyle.

To my literary mentors and friends: Selwyn Seyfu Hinds—thanks for your literary guidance, continuing presence, love, and support. Sharon Green: believing in me, jump-starting my career as an author—I love you dearly. Sam Fine: thanks for all your advice—getting me out of all my sticky situations and most of all that FABULOUS Publicity and Cover Shot!! To Edwidge Danticat for your insight; Colin Channer, Sonia Sanchez, Sonya Allyne, Constance White, and Jill Nelson for all your encouraging words. I pray I haven't forgotten anyone, with love.

Peace and Light Everytime.

Diane

Index

Acuna, Claudia, 164
Aerobic exercise, 32
African Americans, 4
Africans, 4, 20
Afros, xvii, xix–xxi
   in Japan, 87
   metal picks for, 47
Afro Twists, 100, 102
Aguilera, Christina, xix, xxi
Aida (musical), 9
Air drying, 50, 51
Alopecia, 28–31
   traction, 29–30, 61, 136
Anagen stage of hair growth, 18
Androgenic alopecia, 28, 30
Arista Salon and Spa, 87, 102, 162
Ashanti, 153
Asian crème bath treatment, 37, 41
Asians, 4, 6, 20
Aveda hair care products, 20, 23, 27, 40–42, 53,
   77, 90, 103, 104, 106, 114, 115, 134, 147,
   148, 154
Aveeno baby wash and shampoo, 24
Avlon Affirm Fiberguard, 73

Baby Bliss flat iron, 51
Badu, Erykah, 127
Baker, Josephine, 161
Baldness, 28–31
Banks, Tyra, 132
Baptiste, Marc, 89, 159
Barbel, Hadiiya, 102
Barbicide, 45
Bascom, Niya, 163
Beautiful Skin of Color (Cook-Bolden), 25
Beauvais-Nilon, Garcelle, 153
Beliage techniques, 150
BET (Black Entertainment Television), 100,
   102
Bethann Management, xxv, 118, 131

Beyoncé, 151, 152
Bible, 6, 33
Biolage Earth Tones Color Reserve, 42, 154
Blackman, Cindy, 105–7, 152
Blending, 50
Blige, Mary J., 152
Blow-dryers, 45, 50–51
   brushes for use with, 48–50, 77
   cutting and, 66–67
Boar bristle brushes, 48
Bolo, Yami, 120
Bonded weaves, 140–41
Bone combs, 46
Bonet, Lisa, xix
Botanical hair care products, 37, 41, 60, 150
   for relaxed hair, 72
   for weaves, 141
Bounce-back cutting technique, 67
Braids, xvii, xix, xx, xxiii–xxv, xxvii, 10, 81,
   131–38
   African origins of, xix
   to create locs, 121
   hair texture and, 7–9
   in Japan, 87
   in local shops, 60, 61
   revival and retro styles, 136, 137
   of straight hair, 7
   tight, hair loss due to, 29–30, 61, 136
   see also Cornrows
Brandy, xix
Breakage, 27
Breathing techniques, 32
Bridgewater, Dee Dee, 122, 124, 157–58,
   163
Brooklyn Museum of Art, 109
Brother locs, 121
Brushes, 45, 48–49, 77
Buckner, George, 10
Bumble and Bumble, 66, 134
Butterfly clips, 52

Caesars, xxi, xiv, 35, 122, 127, 164
Caribbeans, 4
Carol's Daughter hair care products, 40, 42, 53,
    77, 103, 104, 111, 124, 125, 134
Casamas, xix, 136
Catagen stage of hair growth, 18
Central centrifugal alopecia (CCA), 30
Chapman, Tracy, xxiv
Chemical treatments, *see* Relaxed hair;
    Texturizing
Cherokee, xxiv, 136
Children
    braids for, 134, 145
    chemical hair treatments for, 77–78
    coils for, 146
    healthy hair for, 23–24
    twists for, 147
Chilli, 9
Chopping, 68
Christensen, Kym, 35, 46
Clairol Shimmer Lights Shampoo, 154
Clarifying shampoos, 40
Claws, tortoiseshell, 48
Cleansing shampoos, 40
Clips, 45, 52
Coils, xvii, xxiii, xxiv, 81, 86, 87, 109–15, 148
    for children, 146
    to create locs, 119, 120
    curly, 110
    straw set, 114–15
    twisty, 111–12
Coloring, xxiv, xxvi, 55, 83, 149–58
    chemical treatments and, 75
    conditioning and, 42
    during pregnancy, 153
    seasonal, 59, 149, 150
    tips for, 154
Colorists, 60, 150–52, 154
Combs, 45–48
    cutting and, 66
    thermal, 76
*Complete Book of Essential Oils and
    Aromatherapy* (Woods), 19
Conditioners, 35, 36, 40–42
    for chemically treated hair, 73–76
    color, 154
    combing after applying, 47
    for steaming, 36–39
Conditioning shampoos, 40
Cook-Bolden, Fran, 25, 26, 28, 29
Cornrows, xvii, xix, xxiv, xxv, 86
    extension, 145
    sets, 85, 94, 148
    setting locs with, 121
Cosmicloc, xxi
Curling irons, 45, 52
Curly hair, xvii, xxvi
    blow-drying, 50
    combs for, 46

curling irons for, 52
cutting, 63, 67
locked, 120
natural sets for, 85
see also Loose curly hair; Very curly hair
Cutting, xxvii, 55, 63–69
    style, 65–66

Damaged hair, 35
Dandridge, Dorothy, xix
Dandruff, 24–25
    shampoos for, 25, 40
D'Angelo, 127
Davis, Angela, xxiv
Davis, Michaela Angela, xix, 158
Dawson, Rosario, 8
Deep penetrating conditioners, 38, 41
    for relaxed hair, 74
Dekar Salon, 4
Denise Marie, 123, 124
Denman Brush, 49, 77
Destiny's Child, 153
Diet
    dandruff and, 25
    hair loss and, 27–29, 31
    healthy, 15–18
    split ends and, 27
Dillard, Peggy, xxi
Dirie, Waris, xix
Dr. Bronner's Mild Soap, 24
Dorsey, Chelsea, 148
Dorsey, Leon, 148
Dove hair care products, 40, 41
Dry hair, 35
    dietary causes of, 18
Ducktail clips, 52
Dudley's, 66
Dyaspora Salon and Spa, xxii, 95, 136, 157

East Indians, 4
Eczema, 26
Edo tribe, 87
Egypt, ancient, 109
Elastic bands, 53
Elasticity, 57
Elchim Baby Blss Ionic blow-dryer, 50
Electric barrel curling irons, 52
Emi, 87
Essence magazine, xxi–xxiii, 63, 89, 92, 95,
    102, 110, 156, 160, 163
Essential oils, 19, 42–43
    for steam conditioning, 37–38
Ethiopia, xix
European weave, 140
Eve, 152
Exercise, 32
Extensions, xix, xxiv
    blending, 68
    loc, 120, 121

Face shape, 66
Fades, xxv
Fantail combs, 46, 47
Faulk, Helen Graine, xix
Fekkai, Frédéric, 42
Felipe, 63–64, 71, 73
Finishing products, 43
Flat irons, 45, 51, 67
   for straightening hair, 72–73, 77
Flat twists, xxiv, 85, 86, 94
Follicular degeneration syndrome (FDS), 30
Fowler, Kara, 147
Free natural locs, 120, 121, 147
Fugees, 155
Full Frontal (movie), 114
Fungicidal agents, 25
Fusion weave, 140

G (movie), 113, 114
Gels, 43
   blow-drying and, 51
Genilocs, xxiv, 121
Gentle Treatment, 73, 78
Giovanni, Nikki, xxiv
Girlfriends (TV series), xix
Glosses, 43
Goldwell hair care products, 40, 41, 154
Goodrich, Nanya Akuka, 110
Gordon, Ed, 145
Gordon, Taylor, 145
Graham Webb hair care products, 40, 41, 53
Green, Janine, 110
Greenwood, Glenn, 163
Greenwood, Monique, 163
Grier, Pam, xix
Groove Theory, 9
Growing-out, 64–65, 75
   braids and weaves and, 131
   relaxers, 75–76
Growth of hair, *see* Hair growth
Gunshots in My Cook-Up (Hinds), xxvi

Hair care products, 35–43
   for braids, 134, 135, 138
   for coils, 111
   for locs, 120, 124, 128
   for natural free sets and styles, 90, 93, 96
   for twists, 103, 114
   see also specific products and brands
Hair care specialists, 59–60
Hair designers, 59
Hair growth, 18–19
   ancient recipes for, 20
   during pregnancy, 21–22
Hair loss, 19, 27–31
   after childbirth, 21
   shea butter for, 42
Hairpins, 52
Hair spray, 43

Hardison, Bethann, xxv, 95, 118–19, 131–32
Hardison, Kadeem, 95
Hargrove, Kamala, 164
Hargrove, Roy, 126, 127, 163, 164
Harlem Hospital, 31
Head & Shoulders, 25
Headley, Heather, 9
Heart & Soul magazine, xxii, 159
Herbal hair products, 37, 41, 150
   for braids, 134
   for locs, 120
   for weaves, 141
Highlights, 150
   for silver hair, 154
High Top, 127
Hill, Lauryn, xx, xxiv, xxvi, 155–56, 160
Hinds, Selwyn Seyfu, xxvi
Holiday, Billie, xix
Honey magazine, xix, 158
Hood dryers, 51
Hoodlum (movie), xix
hooks, bell, xxiv, 12, 16
Hormones
   baldness and, 28, 30
   during pregnancy, 21
Horne, Lena, 154
Human hair
   braids and weaves, 133, 139
   loc extensions, 121

Ibo tribe, 87
Individual braids, xxiv
Infusion 23, 134
Infusion weave, 140
Instant conditioners, 40–41
Interlock invisible weave, 140
Issa, Ray, 162
Iverson, Allen, xxvi

Jackson, Janet, xix, 152
James, Oscar, xxiv
Jazz, 163–64
Jessica, 51
Johnson & Johnson baby shampoo and
   conditioner, 24

Kellam, Genieva, 147
Kenya, xviii, 118
Kenya flat iron, 51
Kerasilk, 41
KeraCare hair care products, 40, 41
Kerr, Denise, 45
Keys, Alicia, xix, 7, 133
Khamit Kinks, 134, 162
Kiehl's hair care products, 24, 40, 96, 97
Kinapps hair salon, xxiii, 42
King, Hollis, 164
Kinky hair, *see* Tightly coiled hair
Kizuri curling irons, 52

Knots, xvii, xxv, 94
    Nubian, 85, 87, 89
    setting locs with, 121
    Ubo, 87, 89, 90
Knot weave, 140
Kravitz, Lenny, xxi, 95–96, 105–7, 120
Kravitz, Zoë, 95

Larrieux, Amel, 9
Latch hook, interlocking with, 140
Latinos, 4
Lawson, Dekar, 4
Leave-in conditioners, 35, 36, 39, 41
    blow-drying and, 51
Lewis, Ananda, 8
Lifestyle, 15, 58
    hair loss and, 27, 28
Lisa Elixer hair care products, 41, 111, 112
Locksmyths Hair Groomers, 117, 162
Locs, xvii, xx, xxiii–xxvii, 10, 81, 117–23
    African origins of, xviii–xix
    clips for, 52
    coils as first stages of, 109
    coily curls on, 87
    coloring, 151
    cutting, 68
    extensions, xix, xxi
    free natural, 120, 121, 147
    hair texture and, 7–9
    in Japan, 87
    revival and retro styles, 122–23
    steam conditioning of, 37
Loctitians, 60
Logics hair care products, 156
Loose curly hair, 4–6, 8–9, 11
    acceptance of, 12
    straightening, 72, 75
Lopox shampoo, 25
L'Oréal Keratase Conditioner, 41
Loss of hair, see Hair loss
Lowlights, 150
LTC, 152

Macklin, Pamela, 63
Maintenance program, 16, 17, 35–43
    stylists and, 59
Marcel Barrel Curling Iron, 52
Marcel waves, xix
Mark H., 163
Marley, Bob, 118
Marsalis, Wynton, 127
Martin, Elizabeth L., 144
Mary Mary, 153
Massai Mara tribe, xviii, 118
Master braiders, 60
Master precision cutters, 60, 66
Maxwell, xxi
McCurtis, Henry, 31
Medicated shampoos, 40

Meditation, 32
Menopause, 30
Metal picks, 47
Michelle, 122, 123
Microextension, 140
Micros braids, xxiv
Minerals, 19
Minoxidil, 28–29
Mizani hair care products, 40, 41, 73
Moisturizing conditioners, 41
Moisturizing shampoos, 40
Moods magazine, xxi
Mousse, 43
Mya, 8

Namaska's Muntu Green Drink, 33
Native Americans, 4, 6, 20
Natural free sets and styles, xxvii, 10, 81,
    85–97
    revival and retro, 87–90
Natural hair care specialists, 60
Natural hair salons, 60
Natural Root Organic Stimulator Tea Tree Oil
    Pomade, 128
Natural Uplift Root Stimulator, 40
Neutrogena hair care products, 25, 40, 41, 138
Nigeria, 87
Nizoral shampoo, 25, 26, 40
Normal hair, 35
Nubian knots, 85, 87, 89
Nutrition, 19, 27
    See also Diet

Ogilvie, Peter, 110
Oil treatments, 41
    See also Essential oils
Oily hair, 35
    dietary causes of, 18
Okhura, Phina, 159
Origins hair care products, 40
Osiri Maat, Ona, 109, 117, 162
Oval boar bristle brushes, 48
Overprocessing, 73

Paddle brushes, 48, 50, 77
Pantene Pro-V, 40, 41
Paul Mitchell hair care products, 23–24, 40,
    124, 128
Payton, Nicholas, 164
Peden, Jon, 92
Perimenopause, 30
Phyto hair care products, 27, 28, 40, 41, 93, 138
Picks
    cutting and, 66
    metal, 47
    tortoiseshell, 48
Pinkett Smith, Jada, 152–53
Pirello, Christina, 17–18, 27, 28, 29, 31
Pivot Point, 45, 66

Plaits, 85, 86, 94
    setting locs with, 121
Poe, Deidre, 146
Poetic Justice (movie), xix
Polycystic ovarian syndrome, 30
Pomades, 43
Ponytails, xix, 138, 147
Porosity, 57
Precision cutting, 60, 63, 66
    blow-drying and, 67
    shears for, 49
Pregnancy, 21–22, 144
    coloring hair during, 153
Protein conditioners, 39
Psoriasis, 25–26

Quick Weaves, 139–41

Rastafarians, 118
Razor cutting, 68
Razors, 50
Reconstructing conditioners, 38, 41
Reeves, Diane, 152
Relaxed hair, xix, xxiii, xxiv, 71–74
    curling irons for, 52
    cutting, 64
    drying, 50, 51
    growing out, 75–76, 131
    twisted, 99–100
Retro styles, 83
    braids, 136, 137
    coils, 110–12
    locs, 122–23
    natural, 87–90
    twists, 100–102
Revival styles, 83
    braids, 136, 137
    coils, 110–12
    locs, 122–23
    natural, 87–90, 92–94
    twists, 100–102
Richard, Malonda, 100–102
Rinaldo, 161
Robert Fiance Hair Design Institute, xxii
Roberts, Julia, 114
Rogaine, 28
Rollers, 45
Ross, Tracee Ellis, xix, 9
Round brushes, 48, 50
Rowland, Kelly, 153
Rowley, Cynthia, 45

Salons, 60–61
    consultations at, 56
    directory of, 165–76
    trendy, 55
Sam Wong Salon, 113–14
Samburu people, xviii, 118
Sanchez, Sonia, xxiv

Sanders, Evan Poe, 146
Sassoon, Vidal, 66
Scalp
    clean, 35
    conditioning, 20, 36–37, 42
    disorders of, 24–26
    massaging, 134, 135
Scott, Jill, xxvi
Scrunchies, 53
S-curl pattern, 8, 67, 68, 85, 86, 102
Sea Breeze liquid sanitizer, 45
Seborrheic dermatitis, 24–25
    hair loss from, 29
Selsun Blue, 25
Senegalese twists, xix, xxiv, 99
Sensitive by Nature, 73
Sex and the City (TV series), xxi
Shampoos, 35, 36, 40
    for braids, 134, 135
    for colored hair, 154
    for dandruff, 25, 40
    for eczema, 26
    for locs, 120
Shaping, xxvi, xxvii, 36, 63–69
    shears for, 49
    of split ends, 27
Shea butter, 42
Shears, 45, 49
Sheens, 43
Silky locs, 121
Silver hair, 154
Simmons, Deborah A., 18–19, 22, 24–25, 28, 30
Simmons, Kimora Lee, 7
Sister locs, 121
Sisters of the Yam (hooks), xxiv, 12, 16
Slicing, 50, 60
Smith, Matthew Jordan, 122, 136
SoftSheen•Carson, 73
Sophisticates Black Hair Style and Care Guide,
    123
Soul Food (TV series), 9
Source, The, magazine, xxvi
Spiral rods, 85, 94
Spirituality, 33
    locs and, 117–19
Split ends, 27, 36, 64–66
Standard track weaving, 140
Steam conditioning, 36–39, 41
    for braids, 135
    coloring and, 150
Straight hair, xvii, xxv, xxvi, 4, 6, 11
    acceptance of, 12
    blow-drying, 50, 51
    cutting, 63
    locked, 120, 121
    twisted, 99–100
Strand-by-strand weaves, 140
Straw set coils, 114–15
Stress management, 31–33

Studio 1, 102
Styling combs, 48
Stylists, 55–61
    consultations with, 56–59
"Suga shops," 60
Summer, Cree, 9
Super Salano blow-dryer, 50–51
Synthetic hair braids and weaves, 133–34,
    139

Tamia, 75
Tanzania, 117
Tanzania, xviii, 118
T-Boz, 152
Telogen stage of hair growth, 18, 22
Temple, Shirley, 109
Testosterone, 28, 30
Texture and Tones, 73
Textured locs, 121
Texturized cutting, 68
Texturizing, 8, 55, 64, 74–75, 148
Texturizing shears, 49
Thermal straightening, 76–77
Tightly coiled hair, xvii, xxvi, 4–7, 9, 11
    acceptance of, 12
    blow-drying, 50, 51
    conditioning of, 36
    curling irons for, 52
    cutting, 66–67
    growing out, 76
    natural sets for, 85
Tipping, 150
TLC, 9
Tony & Guy, 66
Tools, 45–53
    for braids, 138
    for coils, 111, 114
    for locs, 124, 128
    for natural free sets and styles, 90, 93, 96
    for twists, 103
    see also specific tools
Tortoiseshell claws, picks, and combs, 48
Traction alopecia, 29–30, 61, 136
Tree braiding, 140
Trimming, 63, 65, 66, 69
Turning Heads Salon, xxi, 127
Tweet, 6, 7
Twist Out, xxi, xxiv, 47, 100, 102–4, 106
Twists, xvii, xx, xxiv, xxv, xxvii, 10, 81, 85, 94,
    99–107
    African origins of, xix
    for children, 147
    to create locs, 120
    flat, xxiv, 85, 86, 94

hair texture and, 7–9
    revival and retro styles, 100–102
    Senegalese, xix, xxiv, 99
    two-strand, 87
Twisty Coils, 110–12
Tyson, Cicely, xix

Ubo knots, 87, 89, 90
Underwood, Blair, xiii–xv, xxi, 113–14
Union, Gabrielle, 153
Universal cut, 69
Updos, 121, 122, 125

Very curly hair, xvii, 4–6, 9, 11, 147
    acceptance of, 12
    blow-drying, 50, 51
    combs for, 46, 47
    curling irons for, 52
    cutting, 66–67
    growing out, 75–76
    locked, 120
Vitamins, 19, 26

Walker, Madam CJ, 15
Water wash, 35–36
Wave Nouveau, 73
Wavy hair, xvii, xix, xxvi, 4–6, 8, 11, 144
    acceptance of, 12
    blow-drying, 50, 51
    conditioners for, 36
    combs for, 46
    curling irons for, 52
    cutting, 63, 67, 68
    growing out, 75
    locked, 120
    natural sets for, 85
Waxes, 43
Weaves, xxiv, xxv, 131–33, 139–41
    blending, 68
Wek, Alek, 9
Wide paddle brushes, 48
Wide-tooth combs, 47, 48, 50
    cutting and, 66
Williams, Serena, 9
Williams, Vanessa, 9
Williams, Venus, 9
Wilson, Cassandra, 14, 152
Woods, Valerie Ann, 19
World Hair show, 107

Yarn loc extensions, 121
Yeast, 24–25, 29

Zenzalia-Helm, Lenora, 158, 163